GOD'S WISDOM

The Pro-State

Chase DuQuesnay
& Dr. EnQi

Amazon

Johnson Lovers bwahahahahaha

CONTENTS

INTRODUCTION

Did God have a ride or die chick? Lol...

Seriously...

Was there a woman in God's life, is the Bible quietly Matriarchal?

Is there a sure fire way to shrink a bad Prostate?

This book is supplemental to the Food Chemistry & Kitchen Chemistry Books! You need those!!!

JOHNSONITIS

"Prostatic calcifications are commonly found in men and are thought to be associated with prostatitis, chronic pelvic pain syndrome, and prostate cancer [1,2]. Previously these calcifications were not considered clinically significant and their presence usually not mentioned in diagnostic imaging reports".

When I said get the BleuMagick, people got mad with me and thought I was capping or frauding just for sales! The specific blend of Seamosses, combined with the Detox Kit.... I am trying to provide you a baseline of inner hygiene in your temple. I have been saying yall yelling Pineal Gland calcification meanwhile... Your Johnson on fire, you using penis pills. People want me to sell them penis pills for a 'QUICK FLIP'. I refuse. We have 'D!@K Pills' but they work for women and children too... **Anabolic Hormone Help** is for everyone in today's over estrogen filled matrix!

When we first made these herbs, it was called Magic Bond. The Magic Bond is the Bond between Lovers and between Parents/Children. You may be thinking that Testosterone and Estrogen have equal wait in today's issues, they do not. It is Estrogen Dominance that is causing Mental and Physical distress. Even with something as small as ambition and drive. Motivational speakers make millions by colonizing estrogen dominant people. They are chronically under motivated, great for return business. You will find that these gurus isolate themselves from their loving people. Why? They are tired of them being needy. Why? They aren't truly built to heal, nor are they offering long term healing solutions. This is why they just create long terms payment plans and programs to match. They are never planning on you healing and moving on. That's not the game, they begin to believe they are special. When they spot a driven person they pull them into the hustle as a true believer. They can help the movement. We have to be better, we have to truly better people, uplift people.

This prostate issue is a issue for all men, the problem is **BLACK MEN**... Harvard has put out the most recent findings, we have 60% more risk of all problems prostate! Why? Godlessness.

Doc are there healthy people that don't believe in God? Yes, healthy-ish. If we strictly measure health in a physical sense, sure there are very healthy people that are Godless. They are religious though, which makes them mentally ill, no matter how well they function in society. The Breath you breath, is intimately tied to all things life and God. A person can not be healthy without training the Breath. A athlete or anyone that works out is religious. In fact most of them will tell you "I workout religiously". Repetitious breath work of any kind is Religion.

Religion - **a particular system of faith and worship**. c. 1200, religioun, "state of life bound by monastic vows," also "action or conduct indicating a belief in a divine power and reverence for and desire to please it," from Anglo-French religiun (11c.), Old French religion, relegion "piety, **devotion**; religious community," and directly from Latin religionem (nominative religio) "**respect for what is sacred**, reverence for the gods; **conscientiousness**, sense of right, **moral obligation**; fear of the gods; divine service, religious observance; a religion, a faith, a mode of worship, cult; sanctity, **holiness**," in Late Latin "monastic life" (5c.).

This noun of action was derived by

Cicero from relegere "go through again" (in reading or in thought), from re- "again" (see re-) + legere "read" (see lecture (n.)). However, popular etymology among the later ancients (Servius, Lactantius, Augustine) and the interpretation of many modern writers connects it with religare "to bind fast" (see rely), via the notion of "place an obligation on," or "bond between humans and gods." In that case, the re- would be intensive. Another possible origin is religiens "careful," opposite of negligens.

In English, the meaning "particular system of faith in the worship of a divine being or beings" is by c. 1300; the sense of "recognition of and allegiance in manner of life (perceived as justly due) to a higher, unseen power or powers" is from 1530s.

Holistic is Holiness. It is crazy to me when you have Holistic Healers that do not discuss God. They will even attempt to debate the Holistic definition and tie it to Whole only... How can you be whole, without reverence for your ancestors? God is just an ancestor. You can idealistically trace your earthly ancestors back to single cells then what? What was the driving intelligence then, before then? God. The easier lower hanging fruit though, Health.

Health - Old English hælþ "**wholeness**, a being

whole, **sound** or well," from Proto-Germanic *hailitho, from PIE *kailo- "whole, uninjured, of good omen" (source also of Old English hal "**hale**, whole;" Old Norse heill "**healthy**;" Old English halig, Old Norse helge "**holy, sacred**;" Old English hælan "to heal"). With Proto-Germanic abstract noun suffix *-itho (see -th (2)).

Of physical health in Middle English, but also "**prosperity**, happiness, welfare; preservation, safety." An abstract noun to whole, not to heal. Meaning "a salutation" (in a toast, etc.) wishing one welfare or prosperity is from 1590s. Health food is from 1848.

You see that in there? Holistic Health includes but is not limited to Holy.

Holy - Old English halig "holy, consecrated, **sacred**; **godly**; ecclesiastical," from Proto-Germanic *hailaga- (source also of Old Norse heilagr, Danish hellig, Old Frisian helich "holy," Old Saxon helag, Middle Dutch helich, Old High German heilag, German heilig, Gothic hailags "holy"), from PIE *kailo- "whole, uninjured" (see health). Adopted at conversion for Latin sanctus.

The primary (pre-Christian) meaning is not possible to determine, but probably it was "**that must be preserved whole or intact**, that cannot be transgressed or violated," and connected with Old English hal (see health) and Old High

German heil "health, happiness, good luck" (source of the German salutation Heil). Holy water was in Old English.

Holy is stronger and more absolute than any word of cognate meaning. That which is sacred may derive its sanction from man ; that which is holy has its sanctity directly from God or as connected with him. Hence we speak of the Holy Bible, and the sacred writings of the Hindus. He who is holy is absolutely or essentially free from sin; sacred is not a word of personal character. The opposite of holy is sinful or wicked; that of sacred is secular, profane, or common. [Century Dictionary, 1895]
Holy has been used as an intensifying word from 1837; in expletives since 1880s (such as holy smoke, 1883, holy mackerel, 1876, holy cow, 1914, holy moly etc.), most of them euphemisms for holy Christ or holy Moses. Holy Ghost was in Old English (in Middle English often written as one word). Holy League is used of various European alliances; the Holy Alliance was that formed personally by the sovereigns of Russia, Austria, and Prussia in 1815; it ended in 1830.
There is nothing more sacred than life itself. This means Holistic Health a in fact a chicken with it's head cut off, without God. Satanist are real too...

Scrupulosity - A mental illness being excessively

concerned about doing things right in God's eyes.

Origin from Scrupulous meaning - mid-15c., "characterized by fine distinctions of doubt," from Anglo-French scrupulus (Old French scrupulos, Modern French scrupuleux) and directly from Latin scrupulosus "careful, exact," from scrupulus (see scruple). By 1540s as "careful to follow the dictates of conscience," hence, in non-moral matters, "exact, precise, rigorous,
punctilious" (1630s). Scruplesome "inclined to be scrupulous" is from 1800 (Maria Edgeworth). Related: Scrupulously; scrupulousness; scrupulosity.

Who would make being careful and exact, or being careful to follow your conscience, a mental illness? How is being careful and exact, or being careful to follow your conscience a mental illness, in a world where a man can identify as a women? Huh?

Orthorexia - A mental illness being overly concerned about avoiding toxic or unnatural food.

Origin from the Greek ὀρθο- (ortho, "right"

or "correct"), and ὄρεξις (orexis, "appetite"), literally meaning 'correct appetite', but in practice meaning 'correct diet'.

Who would make eating the correct diet a mental illness? How is eating the correct diet a mental illness, in a world where a man can identify as a women? Huh?

Get it? The devil is not a red man with horns, or a Whitman in a suit. The Devil is anyone, of any color or creed, that wants to shorten your life, lower the quality of your life, put you in a position to deny the sacredness of life as a whole... That means certain religious zealots or groups of zealots, are Satanists disguised as God lovers.

Deism - the philosophical position and rationalistic theology[5] that generally rejects revelation as a source of divine knowledge and asserts that empirical reason and observation of the natural world are exclusively logical, reliable, and sufficient to determine the existence of a Supreme Being as the creator of the universe.

The Observer Effect - In physics, the observer effect is the disturbance of an observed system by the act of observation.

The problem with outdated views is…

Many of the Rationalist views have not considered deeply two things: Quantum Entanglement & the Observer Effect. Those two things end all discussion about God, gods and religion. In fact, the Bible discuss the principle of smaller gods in one of my favorite verses.

Matthew 18

19 Again I say unto you, That **if two of you shall agree on earth as touching any thing** that they shall ask, it shall be done for them of my Father which is in heaven.

20 **For where two or three are gathered together in my name, <u>there am I in the midst of them</u>**.

These verses are very mystical unless… we take god literally as Waves.

God - Electromagnetic Waves & Mechanical Waves, self organizing waves.

God is the Word and God is Light.

The trinity is Electricity, Magnetism & Light.

When people gather of like minds, they share their light, electricity and magnetism. They literally create magnetic fields of thought. You can actually feel this, in fact you can feel them on a very small level. Vibes. We are hyper sensitive to vibes. The thing you may not know is the more particular frequencies are repeated in a space, the vibe becomes stronger. When you come into a space, 9/10 times the vibe of that space will over take you! This is why mob mentality is a real thing. You just didn't know because Satanis are in control of the flow of information that, that is a two way street. People aren't just dummer in packs, they are smarter in packs. The group frequency is multiplied by the group. Violent place inspires fear and violence, a clean place inspires cleanliness, a power hungry place inspires the hunger for power, a drug using neighborhood inspires drug abuse, PDFile abuse inspires ________, a educated space inspires education, a gym inspires exercise... Why? Breathing together &/or touching create circuits.

Breathing together is very much like fiber optics, touching is very much like copper wires. Sharing Light &/or Electricity, builds magnetic fields around you. These magnetic fields store information, our Opsins and Melanin interpret this information as Vibes, which is close, they are waves. Vibes become Feelings, become biochemistry & thoughts. Ego prevents gathering in harmony, ego is a mental form of Johnsonitis.

Holistic Healers come in three categories, ignorant of what they are doing, God promoting or Satan promoting. The Satan promoters have the largest reach lmao…. (Doc you sure this aint hating)…

If you know that Holistic Healing must include God, and mislead people, what is that?

If you know that Holistic Healing must include God, and lead them into some sort of perversion, what is that?

I have to teach you about Shu or I'd be a hypocrite. People are accusing me of being a Omnist.

Omnism - the belief in all religions.

I am not. I am a Monotheist. I do believe that language causes most confusion, along with Satanist. Satanist intentionally mislead folks. Egyptologist are intentionally misleading folks, if Khufu built the great pyramid, he did not build that out of ego or Johnsonitis.

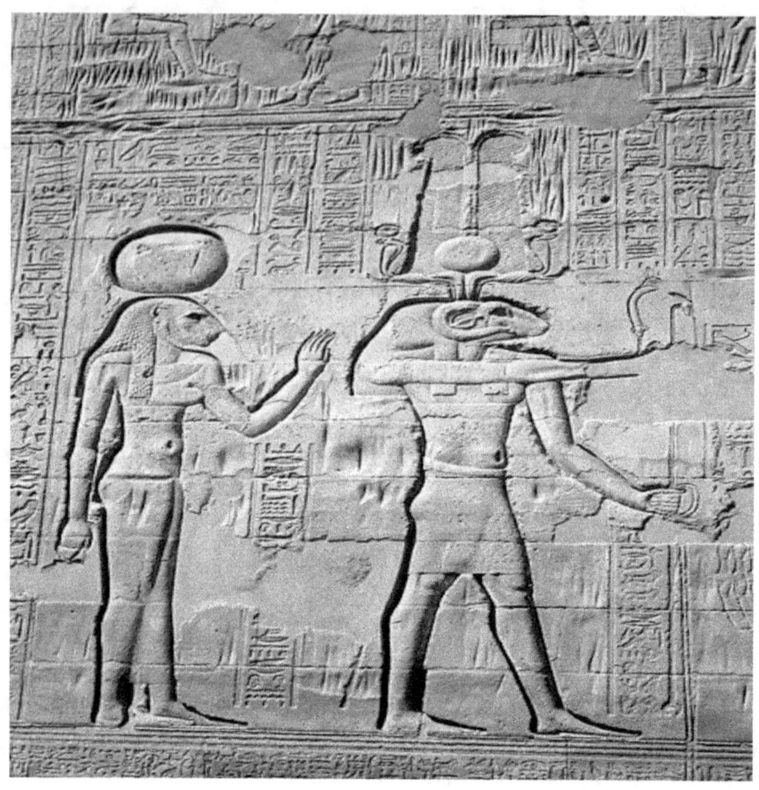

Khufu's full name was Khnum-Khufwy, which means '[the god] Khnum protect me'. His only surviving statue is, ironically, the smallest piece of Egyptian royal sculpture ever discovered: a 7.5 cm (3 inch) high ivory statue found at Abydos. Khnum shapes, Shu supplies the Breath of Life.

Notice that Khnum is wearing the Shu'ty Crown or Double Feather Crown. Khnum got the Antenna on his Crown and his Head, with the Nagas on it. I'm going somewhere with this... The purpose of the small shafts inside the Great Pyramid of Giza is still a mystery. However, there are a number of theories about what they may have been used for. One theory is that the shafts were used for ventilation. The Great Pyramid is a massive structure, and it would have been hot and stuffy inside. The pyramid was sealed and was not meant for people to be in there! That means that theory is dead. The Kings Chamber is entirely lined and roofed with **granite**. From the chamber two narrow shafts run obliquely through the **masonry** to the exterior of the pyramid; it is not known whether they were designed for a religious purpose or were meant for ventilation.... This is also a lie. Geb, Shu & Tefnuit created this 'space' for life. The King's Chamber is meant to be empty or filled with air because that is the King.

Shu is the God of Emptiness and Air, the King is in his Chamber, in his palace at all times. We need to be humble, the meek will inherit the Earth.

This is where we need to pick up because meek isn't sick or weak. We need to worship, as workship, the divine, by working on our Temple. We need to worship, as workship, the divine, by working on our Breath. We need to worship, as workship, the divine, by consuming our Greens. This is the understanding of Wusir as the Earthly manifestation of the Gods, human kind being Green & Black. Chlorophyl and Melanin, eat your Greens. The Pyramid is built with Algae, eat your BleuMagick. The calcification of the prostate is because we have poor muscle development and horrible iodine metabolism.

PROSTATE

Guess What? Chicken Butt! Guess Who? Me and You!

Black men the Prostate goes bad 60% blah blah blah...

Harvard Health Publishing

The prostate gland isn't big—about the size of a walnut—but its location virtually guarantees problems if something goes awry. The prostate gland is located just below the bladder and in front of the rectum. It also wraps around the upper part of the urethra, the tube that carries urine from the bladder out of the body. That means prostate problems can affect urination and sexual function.

The prostate is prone to three main conditions:

Prostatitis: infection or inflammation of the prostate

Benign prostatic hyperplasia (BPH): aging-related enlargement of the prostate gland

Prostate cancer: the growth of cancerous cells inside the prostate, which may break out of the gland and affect other parts of the body.

Prostate function: What does my prostate do?

Your prostate plays a key role in reproduction. Although it's the testicles that produce sperm, the prostate (along with tiny neighboring organs called seminal vesicles) helps produce semen—the viscous fluid in which sperm travel.

Here's what happens when you ejaculate. Within the prostate, a series of ducts lined with fluid-producing cells pushes prostatic fluid out into the urethra (the tube that carries urine from the bladder) where it joins both the sperm produced by the testicles and the fluids generated by the seminal vesicles (narrow glands located on each side of the prostate).

The prostate consists of two lobes, right and left, and it's wider at its base. The base of the prostate is higher up in your body, where the gland nestles against the bladder. The "apex" is the lower end, closer to the rectum. Between the apex and the base lies the mid-gland. These terms are important in discussions about prostate cancer, since the area of the prostate in which a cancer appears can affect symptoms, treatment options and outcomes.

What are common prostate problems?

Unfortunately, most men will experience some kind of prostate problem during their lifetime. Prostate problems are generally associated with three conditions: prostatitis, BPH, and cancer.

Prostatitis refers to an inflamed prostate. There are two main types: acute prostatitis and chronic prostatitis. Acute prostatitis is caused by an infection, usually by bacteria, and results in the sudden onset of painful urination, a small stream and often fever and chills, Chronic prostatitis, also known as chronic pelvic pain syndrome, is a less well defined condition. Its symptoms include persistent or recurrent pelvic discomfort, pain or burning with urination, an increased urge to urinate, difficulty emptying their bladders, and/or painful ejaculation. The underlying cause can be a chronic inflammation with or without an infection, and often the exact reason for symptoms can't be found.

Benign Prostatic Hyperplasia (BPH), commonly called "enlarged prostate," refers to the excessive growth of the gland that usually occurs after age 50; it can double or triple in mass during the latter decades of life. BPH is not caused by cancer (though it can occur alongside it).BPH can be considered an expected part of the aging process for most men. About half of cases are asymptomatic, but some men will experience problems. As the prostate expands in size, it effectively pinches off the urethra (the tube carrying urine from the bladder to the penis), making the muscular walls of the bladder have to work harder and causing problems with urination.

As with other cancers, prostate cancer is the abnormal growth of cells. Prostate cancer can be localized (limited to the prostate itself), regionally advanced (spread to surrounding tissue) or metastatic (spread to more distant sites). Recent years have seen great advancements in prostate-cancer screening, testing and treatment.

What causes prostate problems?

Acute prostatitis is usually caused by a bacterial infection. The exact cause of chronic prostatitis/chronic pelvic pain syndrome is often not discovered. One possibility is that the immune system mistakenly targets the prostate, blasting the gland with inflammatory compounds. Another possibility is bacterial or fungal infections that go undetected by standard testing methods. Certain foods may also trigger symptoms, as might stress and depression, chronic pain conditions, trauma to the genitourinary area, and repeated biopsies.

By far, the greatest risk factor for benign prostatic hyperplasia (BPH), or enlarged prostate, is age. However, prostatitis, a sedentary lifestyle, obesity, high blood pressure and diabetes have all been associated with the condition. And researchers have found correlations between BPH and a diet high in sugar, red meat and refined grains.

No exact cause of prostate cancer has been identified, although genetic defects (either inherited or uninherited) play a key role. Age is an important risk factor, as is family history: Men whose fathers or brothers had prostate cancer are two to three times likelier to get it themselves. Race appears to matter, as well—rates among African Americans are 60% higher than in white men. A diet high in red meat and saturated fats has been associated with increased risk, and obesity is a separate risk factor. Some studies suggest that men who **ejaculate infrequently are at higher risk**. High ejaculation frequency was linked to a decreased risk. Compared to men who reported 4–7 ejaculations per month across their lifetimes, men who ejaculated 21 or more times a month enjoyed a 31% lower risk of prostate cancer. And the results held up to rigorous statistical evaluation even after other lifestyle factors and the frequency of PSA testing were taken into account.

An Australian study of 2,338 men examined the impact of sexual factors on the occurrence of prostate cancer before the age of 70. Like the Harvard research, the Australian investigation evaluated total ejaculations rather than sexual intercourse itself. Like the American men, the Australians who ejaculated most frequently enjoyed a reduced risk of prostate cancer. The effect was strongest for the frequency of ejaculations in young adulthood, even though prostate cancer was not diagnosed until many decades later. Even so, the apparent protection extended to all age groups. In all, men who averaged

4.6–7 ejaculations a week were 36% less likely to be diagnosed with prostate cancer before the age of 70 than men who ejaculated less than 2.3 times a week on average.

Iodine deficiency produces hypercalcemia and hypercalcitonemia in rats

O H Clark, S J Rehfeld, B Castner, J Stroop, H F Loken, L J Deftos

Abstract

To determine the effect of thyroid-stimulating hormone (TSH) on secretion of calcitonin by the thyroid, 50 male Sprague-Dawley rats were randomly separated into seven groups. The groups received different diets, medications, or operations [propylthiouracil (PTU), iodine-deficient diet, (LID), acute or chronic thyroxine treatment, sham operation (SO), hemithyroidectomy (Htx), and total thyroidectomy (Ttx)]. two weeks to six months later, serum TSH concentrations were increased in the Htx, Ttx, and LID groups when compared with SO animals. Serum calcitonin concentrations were increased in the LID- and PTU-treated groups and were decreased in animals that chronically received thyroxine. Serum calcium concentrations were increased in the LID animals, decreased in the Ttx animals, and were similar in the other groups.

These findings suggest that TSH stimulates both follicular and parafollicular cells in the rat thyroid and that iodine deficiency causes hypercalcemia and hypercalcitonemia.

Watch this! Iodine deficiency disorders are the most common cause of preventable brain damage, which affects an estimated 50 million people worldwide. During pregnancy, severe iodine deficiency may impair fetal development, resulting in cretinism (irreversible mental retardation with short stature and developmental abnormalities) as well as in miscarriage and stillbirth. Other more pervasive consequences of chronic iodine deficiency include lesser cognitive and neuromuscular deficits. The ocean is a dependable source of iodine, but away from coastal areas iodine in food is variable and largely reflects the amount in the soil. In chronic iodine deficiency the thyroid gland enlarges as it attempts to trap more iodide (the form in which iodine functions in the body) from the blood for synthesis of thyroid hormones, and it eventually becomes a visible lump at the front of the neck known as a goitre. **Some foods, such as cassava, millet, sweet potato, certain beans, and members of the cabbage family, contain substances known as goitrogens that interfere with thyroid hormone synthesis**; these substances, which are destroyed by cooking, can be a significant factor in persons with coexisting iodine deficiency who rely on goitrogenic foods as staples. This is a problem with Raw foodists, they don't have a complete grip on biochemistry. We don't do Raw Seamoss ever... High intake of vitamin D can lead to a variety of debilitating effects, notably calcification of soft tissues and cardiovascular and renal damage. Although not a concern for most people, young children are especially vulnerable to vitamin D toxicity.

Here is the research...

Molecular iodine (I2) has garnered attention in recent studies for its potential antiproliferative effects and its ability to sensitize various cancer cells to the differentiating effects of retinoic acid. Understanding these mechanisms can provide insights into potential therapeutic strategies in oncology.

Antiproliferative Effects of Iodine

Iodine, particularly in its molecular form (I2), has been observed to exert strong antiproliferative effects on various cancer cell lines. This includes modulation of cell cycle progression and induction of apoptosis, which contribute to reduced cell growth and proliferation. Molecular iodine has been shown to affect mitochondrial function and induce oxidative stress, ultimately leading to cellular death in tumor cells.

Mechanism of Action

The exact molecular mechanisms by which I2 induces antiproliferative effects are still under investigation. However, studies suggest that iodine can disrupt cellular signaling pathways that are essential for cancer cell survival and proliferation, including the modulation of gene expression related to apoptosis and cell cycle regulation. This disruption may enhance the sensitivity of cancer cells to chemotherapeutic agents and other differentiating agents like retinoic acid.

Sensitization to Retinoic Acid Effects

Moreover, iodine has been reported to sensitize cancer cells to differentiating effects when combined with retinoic acid. Retinoic acid (RA), a metabolite of Vitamin A, plays a key role in the regulation of gene transcription, influencing processes such as cell differentiation, growth, and apoptosis. The combined use of I2 and RA may improve the effectiveness of RA therapy, particularly in cancers that display resistance to typical treatments.

Role of Retinoic Acid

Retinoic acid functions by binding to retinoic acid receptors (RARs), leading to alterations in gene expression that promote differentiation and inhibit proliferation. The sensitization by iodine could involve the enhancement of RA's efficacy through various cellular pathways, including antioxidant mechanisms that reduce oxidative damage, thereby allowing RA to act more effectively.

Implications for Cancer Treatment

The potential for molecular iodine to act synergistically with retinoic acid opens avenues for novel therapeutic strategies in cancer treatment. By incorporating I2 into treatment regimens, it may be possible to enhance the therapeutic outcomes of retinoic acid, potentially addressing some of the challenges faced with chemoresistance in certain malignancies. This dual approach suggests that patients may benefit significantly from the combined use of iodine and RA, warranting further clinical investigation.

Conclusion

Molecular iodine demonstrates promising potential in inducing antiproliferative effects and sensitizing cancer cells to retinoic acid. These findings highlight the potential for iodine as a valuable adjunct in cancer therapy, enhancing the effectiveness of existing treatments and providing a basis for further research into its mechanisms and clinical applications. Future studies are essential to better understand the therapeutic implications and the underlying biology of these interactions.

Let me add something here, many egyptologist will tell you, to study politics or war. They will tell you this right after they tell you the meaning of Neter.

Neter (Netjer) - the egyptian word for god by e. a. wallis budge! This is incorrect, it actually means divine &/or vital forces. If you meditate on the meaning of Neter, what would the Gods themselves tell you to study? Life Science, and the cultivation of life. If you don't understand that, you can't truly engage in politics (or war).

Politics - the activities associated with the governance of a country or other area, especially the debate or conflict among individuals or parties having or hoping to achieve power.

The purpose of power and control of resources is to support life and particular lifestyles. The King who built the great pyramid's name is Khnum-Khufwy, which means '[the god] Khnum protect me'. Another important name for our conversation is Djoser Netjerikhet aka the first God Body. This is the real God Body OG!!!

Djoser Netjerikhet - His name Netjerikhet means "divine of body" and 'Djoser' is derived from the Djed symbol of stability. He succeeded his father, Khasekhemwy, the last king of the Second Dynasty, and his mother was the queen Nimaathap. Djoser dispatched several military expeditions to the Sinai Peninsula, during which the local inhabitants were subdued. He also sent expeditions there to mine for valuable minerals such as turquoise and copper. This is known from inscriptions found in the desert there, sometimes displaying the banner of Set alongside the symbols of Horus, as had been more common under Khasekhemwy. The Sinai was also strategically important as a buffer between the Nile valley and Asia. I am also demonstrating that the Sinai was under the banner of Kemet for centuries before Greek colonization. An inscription known as the Famine Stela and claiming to date to the reign of Djoser, but probably created during the Ptolemaic Dynasty, relates how Djoser rebuilt the temple of Khnum on the island of Elephantine at the First Cataract, thus ending a seven-year famine in

Egypt.

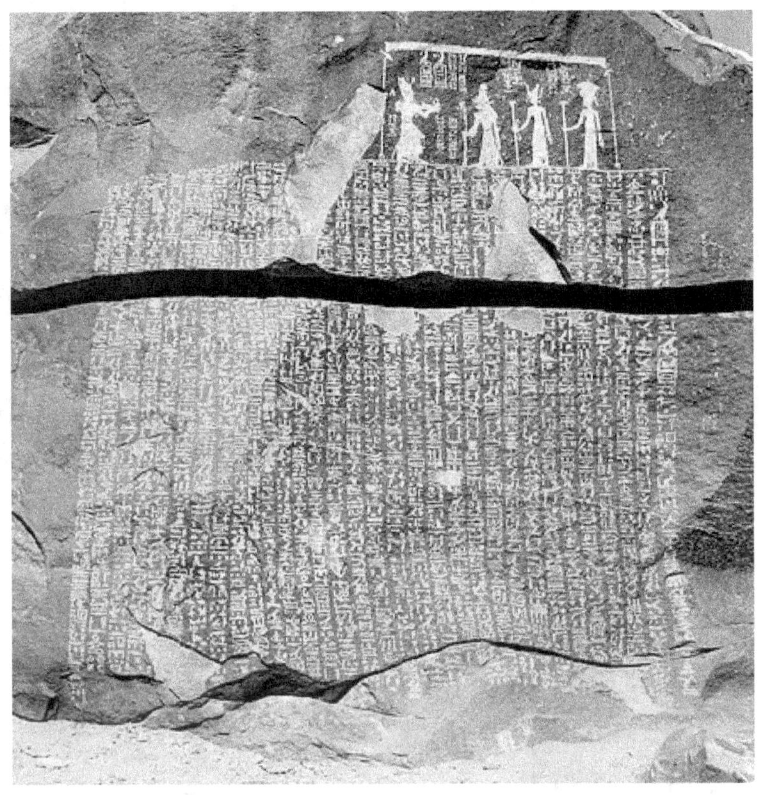

The GodBody is famous for ending the 7 year famine.

Genesis 41

And it came to pass at the end of two full years, that Pharaoh dreamed: and, behold, he stood by the river.

2 And, behold, there came up out of the river seven well favoured kine and fatfleshed; and they fed in a meadow.

3 And, behold, seven other kine came up after them out of the river, ill favoured and leanfleshed; and stood by the other kine upon the brink of the river.

4 And the ill favoured and leanfleshed kine did eat up the seven well favoured and fat kine. So Pharaoh awoke.

5 And he slept and dreamed the second time: and, behold, seven ears of corn came up upon one stalk, rank and good.

6 And, behold, seven thin ears and blasted with the east wind sprung up after them.

7 And the seven thin ears devoured the seven rank and full ears. And Pharaoh awoke, and, behold, it was a dream.

8 And it came to pass in the morning that his spirit was troubled; and he sent and called for all the

magicians of Egypt, and all the wise men thereof: and Pharaoh told them his dream; but there was none that could interpret them unto Pharaoh.

9 Then spake the chief butler unto Pharaoh, saying, I do remember my faults this day:

10 Pharaoh was wroth with his servants, and put me in ward in the captain of the guard's house, both me and the chief baker:

11 And we dreamed a dream in one night, I and he; we dreamed each man according to the interpretation of his dream.

12 And there was there with us a young man, an Hebrew, servant to the captain of the guard; and we told him, and he interpreted to us our dreams; to each man according to his dream he did interpret.

13 And it came to pass, as he interpreted to us, so it was; me he restored unto mine office, and him he hanged.

14 Then Pharaoh sent and called Joseph, and they brought him hastily out of the dungeon: and he shaved himself, and changed his raiment, and came in unto Pharaoh.

15 And Pharaoh said unto Joseph, I have dreamed a dream, and there is none that can interpret it: and I have heard say of thee, that thou canst understand a

dream to interpret it.

16 And Joseph answered Pharaoh, saying, It is not in me: God shall give Pharaoh an answer of peace.

17 And Pharaoh said unto Joseph, In my dream, behold, I stood upon the bank of the river:

18 And, behold, there came up out of the river seven kine, fatfleshed and well favoured; and they fed in a meadow:

19 And, behold, seven other kine came up after them, poor and very ill favoured and leanfleshed, such as I never saw in all the land of Egypt for badness:

20 And the lean and the ill favoured kine did eat up the first seven fat kine:

21 And when they had eaten them up, it could not be known that they had eaten them; but they were still ill favoured, as at the beginning. So I awoke.

22 And I saw in my dream, and, behold, seven ears came up in one stalk, full and good:

23 And, behold, seven ears, withered, thin, and blasted with the east wind, sprung up after them:

24 And the thin ears devoured the seven good ears: and I told this unto the magicians; but there was none that could declare it to me.

25 And Joseph said unto Pharaoh, The dream of Pharaoh is one: God hath shewed Pharaoh what he is about to do.

26 The seven good kine are seven years; and the seven good ears are seven years: the dream is one.

27 And the seven thin and ill favoured kine that came up after them are seven years; and the seven empty ears blasted with the east wind shall be seven years of famine.

28 This is the thing which I have spoken unto Pharaoh: What God is about to do he sheweth unto Pharaoh.

29 Behold, there come seven years of great plenty throughout all the land of Egypt:

30 **<u>And there shall arise after them seven years of famine</u>**; and all the plenty shall be forgotten in the land of Egypt; and the famine shall consume the land;

31 And the plenty shall not be known in the land by reason of that famine following; for it shall be very grievous.

32 And for that the dream was doubled unto Pharaoh twice; it is because the thing is established by God, and God will shortly bring it to pass.

33 Now therefore let Pharaoh look out a man discreet and wise, and set him over the land of Egypt.

34 Let Pharaoh do this, and let him appoint officers over the land, and take up the fifth part of the land of Egypt in the seven plenteous years.

35 And let them gather all the food of those good years that come, and lay up corn under the hand of Pharaoh, and let them keep food in the cities.

36 And that food shall be for store to the land against the seven years of famine, which shall be in the land of Egypt; that the land perish not through the famine.

37 And the thing was good in the eyes of Pharaoh, and in the eyes of all his servants.

38 And Pharaoh said unto his servants, Can we find such a one as this is, a man in whom the Spirit of God is?

39 And Pharaoh said unto Joseph, Forasmuch as God hath shewed thee all this, there is none so discreet and wise as thou art:

40 Thou shalt be over my house, and according unto thy word shall all my people be ruled: only in the throne will I be greater than thou.

41 And Pharaoh said unto Joseph, See, I have set thee

over all the land of Egypt.

42 And Pharaoh took off his ring from his hand, and put it upon Joseph's hand, and arrayed him in vestures of fine linen, and put a gold chain about his neck;

43 And he made him to ride in the second chariot which he had; and they cried before him, Bow the knee: and he made him ruler over all the land of Egypt.

44 And Pharaoh said unto Joseph, I am Pharaoh, and without thee shall no man lift up his hand or foot in all the land of Egypt.

45 And Pharaoh called Joseph's name Zaphnathpaaneah; and he gave him to wife Asenath the daughter of Potipherah priest of On. And Joseph went out over all the land of Egypt.

46 And Joseph was thirty years old when he stood before Pharaoh king of Egypt. And Joseph went out from the presence of Pharaoh, and went throughout all the land of Egypt.

47 And in the seven plenteous years the earth brought forth by handfuls.

48 And he gathered up all the food of the seven years, which were in the land of Egypt, and laid up the food in the cities: the food of the field, which was round

about every city, laid he up in the same.

49 And Joseph gathered corn as the sand of the sea, very much, until he left numbering; for it was without number.

50 And unto Joseph were born two sons before the years of famine came, which Asenath the daughter of Potipherah priest of On bare unto him.

51 And Joseph called the name of the firstborn Manasseh: For God, said he, hath made me forget all my toil, and all my father's house.

52 And the name of the second called he Ephraim: For God hath caused me to be fruitful in the land of my affliction.

53 And the seven years of plenteousness, that was in the land of Egypt, were ended.

54 And the seven years of dearth began to come, according as Joseph had said: and the dearth was in all lands; but in all the land of Egypt there was bread.

55 And when all the land of Egypt was famished, the people cried to Pharaoh for bread: and Pharaoh said unto all the Egyptians, Go unto Joseph; what he saith to you, do.

56 And the famine was over all the face of the earth: and Joseph opened all the storehouses, and sold unto

the Egyptians; and the famine waxed sore in the land of Egypt.

57 And all countries came into Egypt to Joseph for to buy corn; because that the famine was so sore in all lands.

According to Amos famine is also being cut off from communications with God. My question is, if God is forces behind health... What does being cut off from God look like? It looks like leading in all causes of Death!!!

Calcium deposit in arteries is a health concern plaguing many Americans. According to a recent study published in the National Library of Medicine, calcification of the arteries impacts 90% of men and 60% of women over the age of 70. Black women (50.6%) specifically had a higher prevalence of calcification compared with women of other race/ethnicity groups.

We have already mentioned Iodine, now we need to go back to the perfect Black, with the Green Skin. You have Green Skin. The solution to Calcification is Vitamin K2, I have been telling you guys for years, Vitamin D and Vitamin K. Vitamin K picks up calcium and carries it back to your bones where it belongs. Magnesium, flushes excess calcium out of the body. Both nutrients are in greens!

Magnesium & Iodine are both ar

AmericanHealer.Website!!!

Guess what? The so-called toxin or anti nutrient Phytic Acid also lowers calcification! Eat your Greens and Beans! Pulses build and maintain strong pulses.

Pulse - "a throb, a beat, a stroke," especially a measured, regular, or rhythmical beat, early 14c., from Old French pous, pulse (late 12c., Modern French pouls) and directly from Latin pulsus (in pulsus venarum "beating from the blood in the veins"), past participle of pellere "to push, drive" (from PIE root *pel- (5) "to thrust, strike, drive").
Extended usages, of feeling, life, opinion, etc., are attested from early 16c. The figurative use for "life, vitality, essential energy" is from 1530s.

"peas, beans, lentils; the esculent seeds of any leguminous plant," late 13c., puls, from Old French pouls, pous, pols and directly from Latin puls "thick gruel, porridge, mush," which is suspected of being (perhaps via Etruscan), from Greek poltos "porridge" made from flour, or both the Greek and Latin words might be from the same source (compare pollen), which might be a loanword from a non-PIE Mediterranean language or an as-yet-unknown PIE root.

Pollen - 1760 as a botanical term for the fine, yellowish dust that is the <u>fertilizing element of flowers</u> (from Linnæus, 1751), earlier "fine flour" (1520s), from Latin pollen "mill dust; fine flour," which is related to polenta "peeled barley," and probably to Greek poltos "pap, porridge," and Sanskrit pálalam "**ground seeds**," but the ultimate origin is uncertain.

Why does the definition for Pulses recommend checking out Pollen? Pulses fertilize Humans!

What is a bisphosphonate? a class of drugs that prevent the loss of bone density, used to treat osteoporosis and similar diseases. All bisphosphonate drugs share a common phosphorus-carbon-phosphorus "backbone":
The two PO3 (phosphonate) groups covalently linked to carbon determine both the name "bisphosphonate" and the function of the drugs. Bis refers to the fact that there are two such groups in the molecule. Many commercially important compounds are phosphonates, including glyphosate (the active molecule of the herbicide Roundup), and ethephon, a widely used plant growth regulator. Bisphosphonates are popular drugs for treatment of osteoporosis.
Clodronic acid is a bisphosphonate used as a drug to treat osteoporosis.

In biochemistry and medicinal chemistry, phosphonate groups are used as stable bioisosteres for phosphate, such as in the antiviral nucleotide analog, Tenofovir, one of the cornerstones of anti-HIV therapy. And there is an indication that phosphonate derivatives are "promising ligands for nuclear medicine."

The point I am making is we may just want the vegetables and the exercise! You already have the Constitution and Declaration of Independence, please read &/or reread those books!

Pulses, Oatmeal and Meat Products are great sources for Phosphates and Phytic Acids. This is one of the reasons that Pulses are the only food on earth, consumed by all long living people. The more Algae and Pulses you eat, the lower your risk for calcification. You also need to jump up and down and stimulate the PiezoElectroChemistry...

Please read &/or reread the PiezoElectroChemistry book...

<u>What does GodBody mean</u>? The meaning of "Godbody" is simple. It means that you see God when you look at the body of man and that there is no mystery god in the sky.

When most people that are religious hear this, they immediately think, oh they don't believe in God. When many young people interpret that, they feel comfort in being Godless, right up until they find themselves in trouble. Then they are Muslims or Christians. Listen to me, no mystery God doesn't mean, no God. Once you realize you are Quantunly Entangled to God, you can get to know God, by learning more about yourself.

You are the Temple. The skeleton is the Stone, the Living Stone. You must constantly supply pressure to grow and maintain that Stone. You must constantly supply pressure to grow and maintain electric current, the Ankh within you, the Cross within you, the Trinity and Divinity within you.

The research team of June Chan, Sc.D., at UCSF has shown in multiple studies that exercise can help delay or prevent prostate cancer progression. "Aerobic exercise after prostate cancer diagnosis may reduce the risk of prostate cancer recurrence or death by up to **60 percent**." Chan's earlier studies in this field, funded by PCF more than a decade ago, showed a benefit to an hour of jogging six days a week – the level of exercise most of us can't or don't want to sustain. But don't get discouraged! In more recent studies, she and colleagues have been looking at more doable levels of exercise – walking 30 minutes a day, or three or more hours a week, at a brisk pace (3 mph or faster). The brisk pace is important: **One study** found that men who walked three or more hours a week at a brisk pace after diagnosis had a 57 percent lower risk of having prostate cancer recur than men who walked at a slower pace, for less than three hours a week. "It improves energy metabolism, lowers inflammation and oxidative stress, helps boost immunity, and is beneficial for androgen signaling pathways."

We are already supposed to be on a daily walking program though right?

What is BPH? I will show the research then speak…

Benign Prostatic Hyperplasia (BPH) is a common condition characterized by the enlargement of the prostate gland, which typically occurs as men age. This condition is not cancerous but can lead to various urinary symptoms that may significantly affect quality of life.

Overview of Benign Prostatic Hyperplasia

BPH is also known as benign prostatic hypertrophy or benign prostatic obstruction. The prostate is a small gland located just below the bladder, and it plays a role in producing seminal fluid. As men age, the prostate may undergo changes and begin to enlarge, which can constrict the urethra and obstruct the flow of urine.

Symptoms of BPH

The symptoms associated with BPH can vary in severity but commonly include the following:

Frequent Urination: An increased need to urinate, especially at night (nocturia).

Urgency: A sudden and intense urge to urinate.

Weak Urine Stream: Difficulty starting urination or a

weak and interrupted urine stream.

Incomplete Bladder Emptying: A feeling of not being able to fully empty the bladder after urination.

Less common symptoms may include urinary tract infections, blood in the urine, or acute urinary retention, which is the inability to urinate at all.

Causes and Risk Factors

While the exact cause of BPH is not fully understood, it is believed to be related to changes in hormone levels as men age. Factors that may increase the risk of developing BPH include:

Age: BPH is rare in men under 40 and becomes more common after age 50.

Family History: A family history of prostate problems may increase the risk.

Other Health Conditions: Conditions such as diabetes, heart disease, and obesity have been linked to a higher risk of BPH.

Diagnosis of BPH

Diagnosis of BPH usually involves a combination of medical history, physical examination, and specific tests, such as:

Digital Rectal Exam (DRE): A healthcare provider will palpate the prostate through the rectum to assess its size and texture.

Urine Tests: To rule out infections or other urinary concerns.

<u>Prostate-Specific Antigen (PSA) Blood Test: To assess the level of PSA</u>, which may indicate prostate issues.

Treatment Options

Treatment options for BPH depend on the severity of the symptoms and may include:

Watchful Waiting: For mild symptoms that do not affect daily life, regular monitoring may be sufficient.

Medications: Alpha-blockers and 5-alpha-reductase inhibitors are common medications prescribed to alleviate symptoms and reduce prostate size.

Surgical Options: If medications are ineffective or if symptoms are severe, surgical procedures may be considered to remove excess prostate tissue and relieve obstruction.

Conclusion

Benign Prostatic Hyperplasia is a prevalent condition affecting many older men, leading to bothersome urinary symptoms. Effective treatment options are available, and understanding the nature of BPH is essential for managing its impact on health and quality of life. Early communication with healthcare providers can help address symptoms and optimize treatment outcomes.

Natural food is best regarding side effects, many people blindly hunt 5-alpha-reductase inhibitors, they don't get it. 5α-Reductases, also known as 3-oxo-5α-steroid 4-dehydrogenases, are enzymes involved in steroid metabolism. The enzyme is produced in many tissues in both males and females, in the reproductive tract, testes and ovaries, skin, seminal vesicles, prostate, epididymis and many organs, including the nervous system. Specific substrates include testosterone, progesterone, androstenedione, epitestosterone, cortisol, aldosterone, and deoxycorticosterone. Outside of dihydrotestosterone, much of the physiological role of 5α-reduced steroids is unknown. We are messing with stuff we don't understand!!!

Hibiscus Tea: Hibiscus is often used because it possesses diuretic properties, which may help in increasing urine output and reducing the accumulation of crystals in the kidneys. The antioxidants in hibiscus can also aid in overall renal health.

Chanca Piedra Tea: Known as the "stone breaker," chanca piedra (Phyllanthus niruri) has been traditionally used in herbal medicine to help eliminate kidney stones. It may work by reducing crystal formation and aiding in the dissolution of calcium oxalate stones.

Dandelion Tea: Dandelion has natural diuretic properties, which can support kidney function and enhance urine production. This may help in flushing out toxins and preventing stone formation.

Nettle Leaf Tea: Nettle contains various beneficial compounds that may support kidney health. Its diuretic effects can aid in preventing the formation of stones by increasing urine flow and reducing the concentration of stone-forming substances.

Green Tea: Rich in antioxidants, green tea has been suggested to have protective properties against kidney stone formation due to its ability to reduce oxidative stress.

These teas are fire and their impact goes much further than the kidneys! I honestly think a big impact of Tea drinking is, taking the place of other drinks. **Saw Palmetto is cool, its not a cure**! On the other hand African Pygeum is known to shrink swollen prostates.

Pygeum africanum for benign prostatic hyperplasia

Timothy J Wilt 1, Areef Ishani 2

Abstract

Background

Benign prostatic hyperplasia (BPH), nonmalignant enlargement of the prostate, can lead to obstructive and irritative lower urinary tract symptoms (LUTS). The pharmacologic use of plants and herbs (phytotherapy) for the treatment of LUTS associated with BPH has been growing steadily. The extract of the African prune tree, *Pygeum africanum*, is one of the several phytotherapeutic agents available for the treatment of BPH.

Objectives

To investigate the evidence whether extracts of *Pygeum africanum* (1) are more effective than placebo in the treatment of Benign Prostatic Hyperplasia (BPH), (2) are as effective as standard pharmacologic BPH treatments, and (3) have less side effects compared to standard BPH drugs.

Search methods

Trials were searched in computerized general and specialized databases (MEDLINE (1966 to 2000), EMBASE, Cochrane Library, Phytodok), by checking bibliographies, and by contacting relevant manufacturers and researchers.

Selection criteria

Trials were eligible if they (1) were randomized (2) included men with BPH (3) compared preparations of *Pygeum africanum* (alone or in combination) with placebo or other BPH medications (4) included clinical outcomes such as urologic symptom scales, symptoms, or urodynamic measurements. Eligibility was assessed by at least two independent observers.

Data collection and analysis

Information on patients, interventions, and outcomes were extracted by at least two independent reviewers using a standard form. The main outcome measure for comparing the effectiveness of *Pygeum africanum* with placebo and standard BPH medications was the change in urologic symptoms scale scores. Secondary outcomes included change in urologic symptoms including nocturia and urodynamic measures (peak and mean urine flow, prostate size). The main outcome measure for adverse effects was the number of men reporting adverse effects.

Main results

A total of 18 randomized controlled trials involving 1562 men met inclusion criteria and were analyzed. Only one of the studies reported a method of treatment allocation concealment, though 17 were double blinded. There were no studies comparing *Pygeum africanum* to standard pharmacologic interventions such as alpha-adrenergic blockers or 5-alpha reductase inhibitors. The mean study duration was 64 days (range, 30 to 122 days). Many studies did not report results in a method that permitted meta-analysis. Compared to men receiving placebo, *Pygeum africanum* provided a moderately large improvement in the combined outcome of urologic symptoms and flow measures as assessed by an effect size defined by the difference of the mean change for each outcome divided by the pooled standard deviation for each outcome (-0.8 SD [95% confidence interval (CI), -1.4 to -0.3 (n = 6 studies)]). Men using *Pygeum africanum* were more than twice as likely to report an improvement in overall symptoms (RR=2.1, 95% CI = 1.4 to 3.1). Nocturia was reduced by 19%, residual urine volume by 24% and peak urine flow was increased by 23%. Adverse effects due to *Pygeum Africanum* were mild and comparable to placebo. The overall dropout rate was 12% and was similar between *Pygeum Africanum* (13%), placebo (11%) and other controls (8%).

Authors' conclusions

A standardized preparation of *Pygeum africanum* may be a useful treatment option for men with lower urinary symptoms consistent with benign prostatic hyperplasia. However, the reviewed studies were small in size, were of short duration, used varied doses and preparations and rarely reported outcomes using standardized validated measures of efficacy. Additional placebo-controlled trials are needed as well as studies that compare *Pygeum africanum* to active controls that have been convincingly demonstrated to have beneficial effects on lower urinary tract symptoms related to BPH. These trials should be of sufficient size and duration to detect important differences in clinically relevant endpoints and use standardized urologic symptom scale scores.

Beta-Sitosterol is not it... Beta-Sitosterol is good for lowering Cholesterol. Lowering Cholesterol is good for the Prostate.

Deuteronomy 23

He that is wounded in the stones, or hath his privy member cut off, shall not enter into the congregation of the Lord.

Hold this next one is so powerful I may have to pull out the source!

Proverbs 3:7-8

Be not wise in thine own eyes: fear the Lord, and depart from evil.

It shall be health to thy navel, and marrow to thy bones.

Proverbs is that GodBody talk!!!

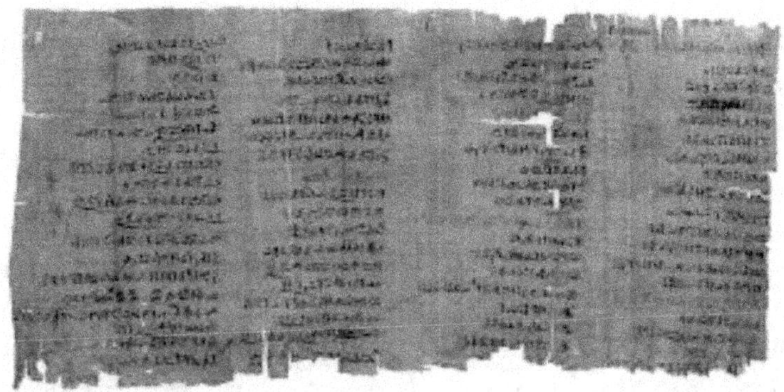

Instruction of Amenemope (also called Instructions of Amenemopet, Wisdom of Amenemopet) is a literary work composed in Ancient Egypt, most likely during the Ramesside Period (ca. 1300–1075 BCE); it contains thirty chapters of advice for successful living, ostensibly written by the scribe Amenemope son of Kanakht as a legacy for his son. It is the culmination of centuries of development going back to the Instruction of Ptahhotep in the Old Kingdom. Egyptian influence on Israel and Judah was particularly strong in the reign of Hezekiah during Egypt's Third Intermediate Period; as a result, "Hebrew literature is permeated with concepts and figures derived from the didactic treatises of Egypt", with Amenemope often cited as the foremost example; the precepts of the Hebrew Bible, and adducing specific parallels between Amenemope and texts in Proverbs, Psalms, and Deuteronomy.

(Proverbs 22:20): "Have I not written for you thirty sayings of counsel and knowledge?"

(Amenemope, ch. 30, line 539): "Look to these thirty chapters; they inform, they educate."

Holistic Healing is a Religion without a head, many people are being mislead into Satanic practices because of this. Anything you do daily is ritual, playing killer games is ritual, eating poison daily is ritual, getting high every day is ritual, watching pornhub daily is a ritual, eating greens everyday is ritual, exercise daily is ritual. What God are you actively serving?

Pastor - late 14c. (mid-13c. as a surname), "**<u>shepherd, one who has care of a flock</u>** or herd" (a sense now obsolete), also figurative, "spiritual guide, shepherd of souls, a Christian minister or clergyman," from Old French pastor, pastur "herdsman, shepherd" (12c.) and directly from Latin pastor "shepherd," from pastus, past participle of pascere "to lead to pasture, set to grazing, cause to eat," from PIE root *pa- "**to feed**; tend, **guard**, <u>protect</u>." Compare pasture.

The spiritual sense was in Church Latin (e.g. Gregory's "Cura Pastoralis"). The verb in the Christian sense is from 1872.

What God are you actively serving? Who is your

Pastor?

Reverend - early 15c., also reverent, "worthy of deep respect, worthy to be revered" due to age, character, etc., from Old French reverent, reverend and directly from Latin reverendus "(he who is) to be respected," gerundive of revereri "to stand in awe of, respect, honor, fear, be afraid of; revere," from re-, here perhaps an intensive prefix (see re-), + vereri "stand in awe of, fear, respect" (from PIE root *wer- (3) "perceive, watch out for").

As a form of address for clergymen, it is attested from late 15c.; earlier reverent (late 14c. in this sense). Prefixed to names by 1640s. Abbreviation Rev. is attested from 1721, earlier Revd. (1690s). Very Reverend is used of deans, Right Reverend of bishops, Most Reverend of archbishops.

Deacon - Middle English deken, "one who reads the Gospel in divine worship, one of a body of assistants to a priest or other clergyman," from Old English deacon, diacon, from Late Latin diaconus, from Greek diakonos "servant of the church, religious official," literally "servant," from dia- here perhaps "thoroughly, from all sides," + PIE *kon-o-, from root *ken- "to hasten, set oneself in motion." Related: Deaconess; deaconship.

Gospel - Old English godspel "**glad tidings announced by Jesus**; one of the four gospels," literally "good spell," from god "good" (see good (adj.))

+ spel "story, message" (see spell (n.1)). A translation of Latin bona adnuntiatio, itself a translation of Greek euangelion "reward for bringing good news" (see evangel).

The first element of the Old English word had originally a long "o," but it shifted under mistaken association with God, as if "**God-story**" (i.e. the history of Christ).

The mistake was very natural, as the resulting sense was much more obviously appropriate than that of 'good tidings' for a word which was chiefly known as the name of a sacred book or of a portion of the liturgy. [OED, 1989]

The word passed early from English to continental Germanic languages in forms that clearly indicate the first element had shifted to "God," such as Old Saxon godspell, Old High German gotspell, Old Norse goðspiall.

Used of anything as true as the Gospel from mid-13c.; as "**any doctrine maintained as of exclusive importance**" from 1650s. As an adjective from 1640s. Gospel music is by 1955. Gospel-gossip was Addison's word ("Spectator," 1711) for "one who is always talking of sermons, texts, etc."

Imam - 1610s, from Arabic, literally "leader; one who precedes," from amma "to go before, precede." As a high religious title used differently by Sunni and

Shiite, but also used of the leader of daily prayers in the mosque and generally for a Muslim prince or religious leader. Related: Imamate.

Rabbi - "**<u>Jewish doctor of religious law</u>**," early 14c. (in late Old English in biblical context only, as a form of address); in Middle English as a title prefixed to personal names, also "a spiritual master" generally; from Late Latin rabbi, from Greek rhabbi, from Mishnaic Hebrew rabbi "my master."

This is formed from -i, first person singular pronominal suffix, + rabh "master, great one," title of respect for Jewish doctors of law. This is from the Semitic root r-b-b "to be great or numerous" (compare robh "multitude;" Aramaic rabh "great; chief, master, teacher;" Arabic rabba "was great," rabb "master").

Minister - c. 1300, "man consecrated to service in the Christian Church, **<u>an ecclesiastic</u>**;" also "an agent acting for a superior, one who acts upon the authority of another," from Old French menistre "**<u>servant</u>**, valet, member of a household staff, administrator, **<u>musician</u>**, minstrel" (12c.) and directly from Latin minister (genitive ministri) "inferior, servant, priest's assistant" (in Medieval Latin, "priest"), from minus, minor "less," hence "subordinate" (from PIE root *mei- (2) "small") + comparative suffix *-teros. Formed on the model of magister (see master (n.)).

Minister views a man as serving a church; pastor views him as caring for a church as a shepherd cares for sheep; clergyman views him as belonging to a certain class; divine is properly one learned in theology, a theologian; parson, formerly a respectful designation, is now little better than a jocular name for a clergyman; priest regards a man as appointed to offer sacrifice. [Century Dictionary, 1895]

The political sense of "high officer of the state, person appointed by a sovereign or chief magistrate of a country as the responsible head of a department of the government" is attested from 1620s, from notion of "**one who renders official service service to the crown**." From 1709 as "a diplomatic representative of a country abroad." A minister without portfolio (1841, in a French context) has cabinet status but is not in charge of a specific department.

An ecclesiastic? Ecclesiastes is from Ptah-Hotep and means public speaking or speaking to the public.

Congregation - late-14c., congregacioun, "a gathering, **assembly**, a crowd; an organized group, as of a religious order or **body of scholars**; act of congregating," from Old French congregacion (12c., Modern French congrégation) and directly from Latin congregationem (nominative congregatio) "an assembling together, union, society," noun of action from past-participle stem of congregare "to herd together, collect in a flock, swarm; assemble," from assimilated form of com "together" (see con-) + gregare "to collect into a flock, gather," from grex (genitive gregis) "a flock" (from PIE root *ger- "to gather").

Used by Tyndale (1520s) to translate Greek ekklesia in New Testament in the sense "an assembly of persons for religious worship and instruction," also "the Christian church in general." The word also was used by Wycliffe and other Old Testament translators in place of synagoge on the notion of "the whole body of the Hebrews, as a community, gathered and <u>set apart for the service of God</u>. (Vulgate uses a variety of words in these cases, including congregatio but also ecclesia, vulgus, synagoga, populus.) Protestant reformers in 16c. used it in place of church; hence the word's main modern sense of "local society of believers" (1520s).

We established that Jewish is Shuish, we have also established that religious law is Mental & Physical Health, with a splash of Abundance. Your Personal Trainer, Holistic Health Teacher, Nutritionist, Herbalist, Doctor etc... is a Rabbi, also worthy of reverence, by going before you, reading the law to and studying the law with you... She or he is shepherding you, where are you going? I know for a fact my Johnson is working! I don't have Johnsonitis lol... I appear before the Lord with proof I have multiplied!!! You better multiply or adopt some babies.... I doing long range adoptions all day.. LOL!!! Seriously though some of you have been surrogate parents to my babies, so you good wether you have babies or not! See and the rest of the family, next time we 'go live'.

Quick Question... Does a Quantumly Entangled group need to be together, to be together? _____.

Doc, what about water?

Drinking less water (or fluid in general) to lessen the symptoms of BPH is no good and may cause more problems than it's worth. It's like diabetes, if you gotta pee, just get up and go pee! Don't stop your water though, unless you have kidney issues. Be mindful of Tap Water, your Tap may be killing you &/ or causing Johnsonitis!

Please go read &/or reread the 40 Day Fruit Fast book!!!!

Quick Question... Did God have a 'Wisdom' with him when he created the World? Was God a Mason?

Proverbs 8

Doth not wisdom cry? and understanding put forth

her voice?

2 She standeth in the top of high places, by the way in the places of the paths.

3 She crieth at the gates, at the entry of the city, at the coming in at the doors.

4 Unto you, O men, I call; and my voice is to the sons of man.

5 O ye simple, understand wisdom: and, ye fools, be ye of an understanding heart.

6 Hear; for I will speak of excellent things; and the opening of my lips shall be right things.

7 For my mouth shall speak truth; and wickedness is an abomination to my lips.

8 All the words of my mouth are in righteousness; there is nothing froward or perverse in them.

9 They are all plain to him that understandeth, and right to them that find knowledge.

10 Receive my instruction, and not silver; and knowledge rather than choice gold.

11 For wisdom is better than rubies; and all the things that may be desired are not to be compared to it.

12 I wisdom dwell with prudence, and find out knowledge of witty inventions.

13 The fear of the Lord is to hate evil: pride, and arrogancy, and the evil way, and the froward mouth, do I hate.

14 Counsel is mine, and sound wisdom: I am understanding; I have strength.

15 By me kings reign, and princes decree justice.

16 By me princes rule, and nobles, even all the judges of the earth.

17 I love them that love me; and those that seek me early shall find me.

18 Riches and honour are with me; yea, durable riches and righteousness.

19 My fruit is better than gold, yea, than fine gold; and my revenue than choice silver.

20 I lead in the way of righteousness, in the midst of the paths of judgment:

21 That I may cause those that love me to inherit substance; and I will fill their treasures.

22 The Lord possessed me in the beginning of his way, before his works of old.

23 I was set up from everlasting, from the beginning, or ever the earth was.

24 When there were no depths, I was brought forth; when there were no fountains abounding with water.

25 Before the mountains were settled, before the hills was I brought forth:

26 While as yet he had not made the earth, nor the fields, nor the highest part of the dust of the world.

27 When he prepared the heavens, I was there: when he set a compass upon the face of the depth:

28 When he established the clouds above: when he strengthened the fountains of the deep:

29 When he gave to the sea his decree, that the waters should not pass his commandment: when he appointed the foundations of the earth:

30 Then I was by him, as one brought up with him: and I was daily his delight, rejoicing always before him;

31 Rejoicing in the habitable part of his earth; and my delights were with the sons of men.

32 Now therefore hearken unto me, O ye children: for blessed are they that keep my ways.

33 Hear instruction, and be wise, and refuse it not.

34 Blessed is the man that heareth me, watching daily at my gates, waiting at the posts of my doors.

35 For whoso findeth me findeth life, and shall obtain favour of the Lord.

36 But he that sinneth against me wrongeth his own soul: all they that hate me love death.

If Proverbs is Kemetic, is wisdom Ma'at?

The Nation of Gods and Earths' Supreme Wisdom states: "Wisdom is the Original Woman because life is continued through her cipher (womb)."

Enough is enough, it's clear now! Eve, SaRaH and now Maa'T... The Bible is clearly Matriarchal.

Sidebar

In males, T and its two metabolites, E2 and DHT, all appear to enhance the development of amygdala-kindled seizures. I can't say a happy wife equals a happy life but... Watch that Almond Joy! The cause for enlarged Prostate though, with all seriousness must be semen. Men who have had their testicles removed at a young age (for example, as a result of testicular cancer) do not develop BPH. When you combine that with the fact that men who ejaculate more often…

Yes… Balance is required, this is not a license to go crazy with Handgela or Palmela, digital porn is very close to sex with a computer. Careful.

Last thing about that Monthly Detox Kit that you don't do every month!!!

NRF2-MEDIATED MACROPHAGE FUNCTION IN BENIGN PROSTATIC HYPERPLASIA: NOVEL MOLECULAR INSIGHTS AND IMPLICATIONS

Guanhui Song a

Jinlin Tong b

Yuhe Wang b

Yuanyuan Li b

Zeqi Liao b

Danping Fan b

Xinrong Fan a b

This article reviews the Nrf2 signaling - mediated macrophage activation mechanism on the BPH immune microenvironment.

The Nrf2 signaling mediates macrophage activation and inhibits BPH by inhibiting pro-inflammatory factors.

The Nrf2 signaling mediates macrophage activation and inhibits BPH by inhibiting oxidative stress disorders.

The Nrf2 signaling mediates macrophage activation and inhibits BPH by initiating apoptosis.

The traditional Chinese medicine based on Nrf2 were summarized to provide ideas for the BPH treatment.

One of the most common urological diseases is benign prostatic hyperplasia (BPH), with a high prevalence in the middle-aged and elderly male population. Patient's mental and physical health is affected significantly by this condition, causing them considerable discomfort. During the development of BPH, a synergistic effect occurs in response to inflammation, oxidative stress, and apoptosis induced by the activation of macrophages. The nuclear factor erythroid2-related factor 2 (Nrf2) signaling pathway can mediate macrophage activation and inhibit prostate hyperplasia by suppressing pro-inflammatory factors, anti-oxidative stress disorder, and initiating apoptosis. The purpose of this study was to review the mechanism of action of Nrf2 signaling pathway-mediated macrophage activation on the immune microenvironment of BPH and to summarize the Chinese medicine based on Nrf2 to provide an overview of BPH treatment options.

Yep… It's long article, that basically says, the Herbs that activate that good ole NRF2 system, can do the trick…

FYI we use African Pygeum in the Detox Kit but for prostates issues, I would take capsules and drink teas! On the flip side, you should be in prevention mode especially if you don't want fingers in your booty!!!

Lastly you have to know, all alcohol, Dairy and Meats are bad for your Pro-State.

Pro - 1866 as a shortening of professional (n.). The adjective is attested by 1915 (in golfing's pro shop, workshop run by the resident professional at a club). The use of professional in reference to prostitutes seems to have accounted for proette in sports writing for "female pro golfer" (1968).

"a consideration or argument in favor," c. 1400, from Latin pro (prep.) "on behalf of, in place of, before, for, in exchange for, just as" (from PIE root *per- (1) "forward," hence "in front of, before, first, chief"). Pro and con is short for pro and contra (c. 1400) "for and against" (Latin pro et contra).
word-forming element meaning "forward, forth, toward the front" (as in proclaim, proceed); "beforehand, in advance" (prohibit, provide); "taking care of" (procure); "in place of, on behalf of" (proconsul, pronoun); from Latin pro (adv., prep.) "on behalf of, in place of, before, for, in exchange for, just as," which also was used as a first element in compounds and had a collateral form por-.
Also in some cases from cognate Greek pro "before, in front of, sooner," which also was used in Greek as a prefix (as in problem). Both the Latin and Greek words are from PIE *pro- (source also of Sanskrit pra- "before, forward, forth;" Gothic faura "before," Old English fore "before, for, on account

of," fram "forward, from;" Old Irish roar "enough"), extended form of root *per- (1) "forward," hence "in front of, before, toward, near," etc.

The common modern sense of "in favor of, favoring" (pro-independence, pro-fluoridation, pro-Soviet, etc.) was not in classical Latin and is attested in English from early 19c.

State - [mode or form of existence] c. 1200, stat, "circumstances, position in society, temporary attributes of a person or thing, conditions," from Old French estat "position, condition; status, stature, station," and directly from Latin status "a station, position, place; way of standing, posture; order, arrangement, condition," figuratively "standing, rank; public order, community organization."

This is a noun of action from the past-participle stem of stare "to stand" (from PIE root *sta- "to stand, make or be firm"). Some Middle English senses are via Old French estat (French état; see estate). The Latin word was adopted into other modern Germanic languages (German, Dutch staat) but chiefly in the political senses only.

The meanings "physical condition as regards form or structure," "particular condition or phase," and "condition with reference to a norm" are attested from c. 1300. The meaning "mental or emotional condition" is attested from 1530s (the phrase state of mind is attested by 1749); the specific colloquial sense of "an agitated or perturbed condition" is from

1837.
The meaning "splendor of ceremony, etc., appropriate to high office; dignity and pomp befitting a person of high degree" is from early 14c. Hence to lie in state "be ceremoniously exposed to view before interment" (1705) and keep state "conduct oneself with pompous dignity" (1590s).

He [the President] shall from time to time give to the Congress Information of the State of the Union, and recommend to their Consideration such Measures as he shall judge necessary and expedient. [U.S. Constitution, Article II, Section iii]

Sense in quantum physics is by 1913.

1590s, "to set in a position, fix (a date, etc.)," from state (n.1) "circumstances, position." The sense of "declare, recite, set down in detail in words" is attested by 1640s from the notion of "placing" the words on the record. Related: Stated; stating.

"political organization of a country; supreme civil power, the government; the whole people considered as a body politic," 1530s, from special use of state (n.1); this sense grew out of the meaning "condition of a country" with regard to government, prosperity, etc. (late 13c.), from Latin phrases such as status rei publicæ "condition (or existence) of the republic."

The sense of "a semi-independent political entity

under a federal authority, one of the bodies politic which together make up a federal republic" is from 1774. The British North American colonies occasionally were called states as far back as 1630s.

State rights in U.S. political sense is attested from 1798 (the form states rights is recorded by 1824): the doctrine that states retain all rights and privileges not delegated to the federal government in the Constitution, in its extreme form including the power and right of sovereignty.

Often contrasted with ecclesiastical power in phrase church and state (1580s). State socialism attested from 1850 as "a scheme of government favoring enlargement of state functions as the directest way to achieve socialist goals."

PROSTATIC CALCIFICATIONS: QUANTIFYING OCCURRENCE, RADIODENSITY, AND SPATIAL DISTRIBUTION IN PROSTATE CANCER PATIENTS

Saurabh Singh a,1,*, Eleanor Martin b,c,1, Henry FJ Tregidgo c, Bradley Treeby c, Steve Bandula a

Highlights

- Intraprostatic calcifications are under-recognized and under-reported in imaging.

- Intraprostatic calcifications are common in patients with prostate cancer.

- They commonly occur within tumors or in the vicinity of tumors.

Keywords: Prostate MRI, Calcification, HIFU, Radiotherapy, Prostate cancer, PSMA PET

Abstract

Background

To evaluate the prevalence, density, and distribution of prostate calcification in patients with prostate cancer.

Methods

Patients who underwent both Gallium-68 PSMA PET/CT and MRI of the prostate over the course of a year were selected for analysis. The CT images with visible calcifications within the prostate were included and calcifications automatically isolated using a threshold of 130 HU. The corresponding multiparametric MRI was assessed and the peripheral zone, transition zone, MRI-visible tumor, and urethra manually contoured. The contoured MRI and CT images were registered using rigid registration, and calcifications mapped automatically to the MRI contours.

Results

A total of 85 men (age range 50–88, mean 69 years, standard deviation 7.2 years) were assessed. The mean serum Prostate Specific Antigen PSA was 16.7, range 0.12 to 94.4. Most patients had intermediate-risk disease (68%; Gleason grade group 2 and 3), 26% had high-risk disease (Gleason grade group 4 and 5), and 6% had low-risk disease (Gleason grade group 1). Forty-six patients out of 85 (54%) had intraprostatic calcification. Calcification occurred more in transition zone than the peripheral zone (65% vs. 35%). The mean density of the calcification was 227 HU (min 133, max 1,966 HU). In 12 patients, the calcification was within an MRI-visible tumor, in 24 patients, there were calcifications within a 9 mm distance of the tumor border, and in 9 patients, there were calcifications located between the urethra and tumor.

Conclusions

Calcifications are common in patients with prostate cancer. Their density and location may make them a significant consideration when planning treatment or retreatment with some types of minimally invasive therapy.

Graphical abstract

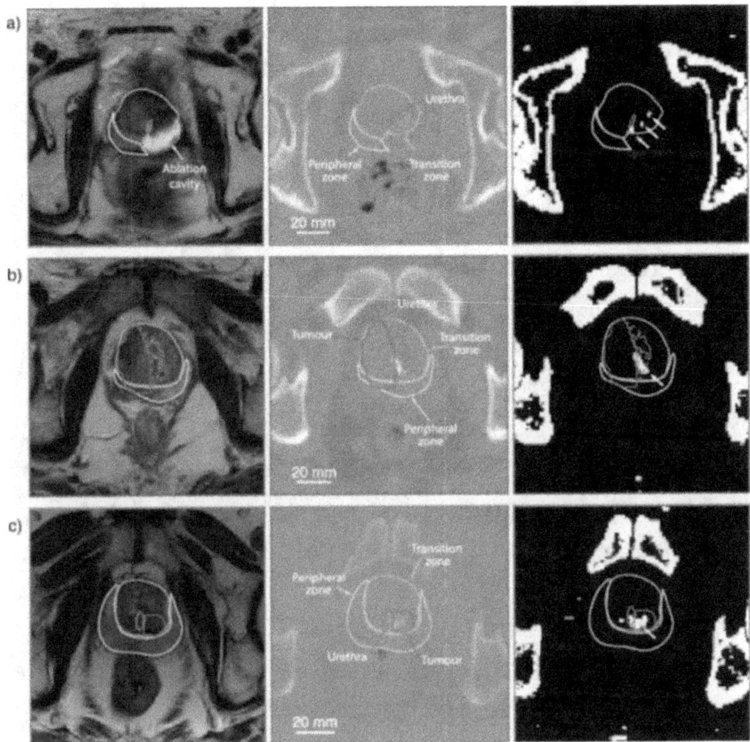

Open in a new tab

1. Introduction

Prostatic calcifications are commonly found in men and are thought to be associated with prostatitis, chronic pelvic pain syndrome, and prostate cancer [1,2]. Previously these calcifications were not considered clinically significant and their presence usually not mentioned in diagnostic imaging reports. Recent studies have however shown that high-density material such as calcification can have a significant impact on treatment delivery in high intensity focused ultrasound (HIFU), transurethral ultrasound ablation, and brachytherapy [3], [4], [5], [6]. In ultrasound therapy, the high-density inclusions can cause reflections of the ultrasound beam, causing changes in the treated volume, which can result in over or under treatment [4,5]. In brachytherapy, the presence of prostatic calcification changes the tissue effective atomic number, leading to altered dose distribution and potential underdosing [3]. Improved understanding of the formation, composition, and distribution of these calcifications could allow development of treatment strategies which mitigate these effects.

The pathogenesis of prostate calcification is thought to be related to prostatic inflammation, urinary retention, or prostatic reflux [7], [8], [9]. These factors are also thought to have a role in prostate cancer and therefore it is not surprising that calcifications coexist in prostates with cancer. The source of calcification is thought to be desquamated acinar cells which form a substance called corpora amylacea. Hydroxyapatite (HA) is then deposited on corpora amylacea forming corporal calculi [7]. An alternative mechanism of HA deposition has been proposed by a group who suggest that HA is deposited by osteoblast-like epithelial cells. The authors suggest that osteoblast-like epithelial cells may be associated with prostate cancer cells and prostate calcification may be a prognostic marker [10].

A few studies have investigated the prevalence of prostate calcification using either imaging or histopathological analysis. A histological study analyzed 298 consecutive whole mount prostate for patients with prostate cancer and found 88.6% contained calcifications [11]. A lower incidence of 58.8% was reported in a study of patients undergoing transrectal sonography who had prostate cancer on biopsy [12]. However, no studies have accurately mapped the location and distribution of calcifications or analyzed their radiodensity using modern CT and MRI. Furthermore, there has been no investigation of calcifications in patients who have undergone treatments such as brachytherapy, HIFU, transurethral ultrasound ablation, or cryotherapy.

The aim of this study was to accurately map and quantify prostatic calcifications using multimodal imaging and computational tools, in a cohort of patients undergoing or having previously undergone treatment for prostate cancer.

2. Materials and methods

Ethical approval for this study was granted by the Yorkshire and the Humber Research Ethics Committee (18/YH/0411).

2.1. Study cohort

In order to select patients who had contemporaneous CT and MRI imaging data, a consecutive cohort of patients who underwent Gallium-68 PSMA PET/

CT and multiparametric MRI (mpMRI; within 6 months of each other) between August 2017 and August 2018 were retrospectively selected. The clinical indications for PSMA PET at our institution are mainly staging of high-risk prostate cancer and assessment of cancer recurrence after treatment. Patients who had a diagnosis of prostate cancer mentioned in the clinical indications were included. Patients who had undergone radical prostatectomy were excluded. Clinical records of selected patients were reviewed for clinical data including PSA and histopathological reports.

2.2. Imaging

A total of 85 datasets were obtained from patients who had undergone both Gallium-68 PSMA PET/CT and MR scans. The whole body CT was acquired with 2.5 mm slice thickness and the modal in-plane resolution was 0.98 mm (min 0.98 mm, max 1.37 mm). The mpMRI included T2W small field of view images, high b-value diffusion weighted imaging (DWI) image (b1400 or b2000), apparent diffusion coefficient (ADC) map, and dynamic contrast-enhanced images. The modal in-plane resolution for the MR images was 0.39 mm (min 0.35 mm, max 0.78 mm) and the modal slice separation was 3.3 mm (min 3 mm, max 3.85 mm). The CT images for all patients were assessed by a Board-certified Radiologist (S.S.).

2.3. Computational analysis

Of these datasets, the prostate and urethra were

contoured on the MR images of 45 datasets, chosen as calcifications were evident on visual inspection of the CT scans. The peripheral and transition zone base, midgland, and apex regions of the prostate, as well as the urethra were contoured by a radiologist, slice by slice using Horos (horosproject.org), then exported as .xml files for further use. Signal abnormality considered as suspicious or highly suspicious for tumor (Likert score 4 or 5) was contoured if it corresponded to cancerous regions on biopsy.

Identification of calcifications was automated in order to reduce variability and increase accuracy of the output statistics. Registration of the CT and MR datasets was performed to allow translation of the contours from the MR images to the CT image space [13], where calcifications can be identified by their radiodensity. For identification of the calculi, the CT images were thresholded at 130 HU. This threshold was selected based on published literature and visual inspection to minimize the detection of noise and beam hardening artifact [14,15]. Each of the contours was defined as a search region, in addition to 3 further search regions. The first of these was derived from the tumor region, grown radially by 9 mm, which is the recommended treatment margin for focal therapy in the prostate [16]. Another region was defined as the volume located between the urethra and tumor search regions. The final region was formed from the sum of all search regions. For each of these regions, clusters of voxels with intensities above the threshold were identified computationally.

For each cluster, the coordinates of the centroid, cluster volume, principal axes lengths of an ellipsoid fitted to the cluster, and mean voxel intensities were computed. Any clusters containing a single voxel were rejected as they were usually found to have voxel intensities close to the threshold, and were indistinguishable from noise on visual inspection. The lateral (in-plane) distance of the centroid of each cluster from the centroid of the urethra search region was also calculated, where the centroid of the urethra was calculated from the mean of the in-plane centroid coordinates across all image slices containing the urethra contour. For each patient, mean, minimum, and maximum values of these quantities were calculated for each contoured region of interest. Calcifications spanning multiple regions of interest were counted in each region. Their statistics were computed only for the part of the calcification located inside each of the zones; the statistics of the entire calcification were computed under the total prostate region, provided it lay fully within that region.

3. Results

3.1. Patient cohort

A total of 85 men (age range 50–88, mean 69 years, standard deviation 7.2 years) were assessed.

The mean PSA was 16.7 ng/ml, range 0.12 to 94.4, standard deviation 19.8. All patients had a diagnosis of prostate cancer and for 78 patients biopsy information was available in their electronic health records. In terms of Gleason grade group; 68% had intermediate-risk disease (Gleason grade group 2 and 3), 26% had high-risk disease (Gleason grade group 4 and 5), and 6% had low-risk disease (Gleason grade group 1). Overall Gleason grade is given in Table 1. Forty-eight patients in this cohort had a history of a previous treatment. Sixteen patients had previous HIFU, 16 had previous external beam radiotherapy, 7 had previous brachytherapy, 3 had previous cryotherapy, 1 had previous chemotherapy, and 1 had reversible electroporation. Some patients had more than one treatment type; 2 had external beam radiotherapy and salvage HIFU, 1 had brachytherapy and salvage HIFU, and 1 had HIFU and cryotherapy.

3.2. Prostate calcification

Intraprostatic calcifications were found in 46 out of 85 patients (Table 2). Examples of corresponding MR and CT images, with visible calculi within transformed region contours, are shown in Fig. 1. An average of 5 foci of calcifications was identified in each patient, with 24 being the highest number of calcifications identified in a single patient. All calcifications were located within 36.9 mm of the centroid of the urethra contour/region of interest (ROI), at a mean distance of 12.1 mm. Calcifications were distributed throughout the regions of the prostate, on average across 4 different regions. The mean volume of calcifications was 55.3 mm^3. The largest calcification, with a volume of 1,263.6 mm^3 spanned several ROIs; it is therefore recorded under the "all regions" search volume, whereas for that patient, the largest calcification found in any region individually had a volume of 689.0 mm^3. This represents only part of the calcification which extends beyond the boundary of this region of interest; a similar occurrence can be observed in Fig. 1A. Most calcifications tended more toward ellipsoid rather than spherical in shape, with a mean aspect ratio of 1:0.74:0.49. Results are shown in for calcifications found in the total region mask and for each ROI individually (Table 2).

Number of calcifications, distance from the urethra, volume, and mean pixel intensity are given as mean (minimum, maximum) of the values for each patient. The distance from the urethra is defined as the in-plane straight line distance between the centroid of the calcification and centroid of the urethra region, where the centroid of the urethra is calculated from the mean of the in-plane centroid coordinates across all image slices containing the urethra contour. PZ = peripheral zone; TZ = transition zone.

Fig. 1.

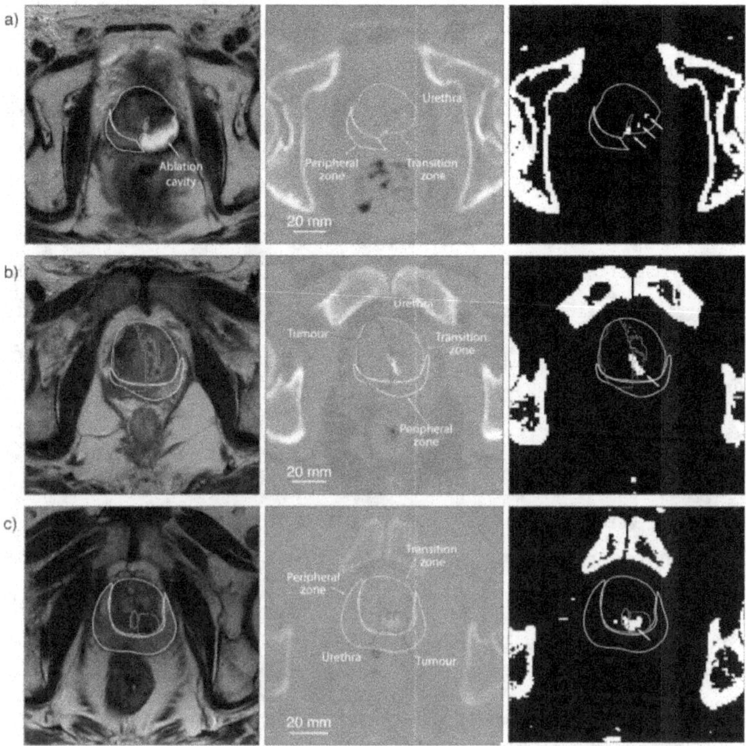

Open in a new tab

T2-weighted MR image slice (left), the corresponding CT image slice (middle), and thresholded image (right) for 3 example cases: (A) previous left-sided HIFU on which calcifications (highlighted by white arrows) are visible within the transition zone midgland contour (blue). (B) Calcification is visible between the urethra and tumor. (C) Calcification is present within the tumor. The peripheral zone midgland (blue), urethra (purple), tumor (red), and area between urethra and tumor (purple dotted) are also shown. (Color version of figure is available online.)

In 33 out of these 46 patients, a MRI-visible tumor was identified. In 12 patients, there were calcifications within the tumor (see Fig. 1C), and 24 patients had calcifications within a 9 mm border of the tumor (see Fig. 1B). In patients with a previous history of treatment, 24 out of 48 (50%) had prostate calcification. In treatment-naive patients, 22 out of 37 (59%) had prostate calcification. There was no statistically significant difference the 2 groups ($P=$ 0.51, Fisher's exact test 2-tailed).

4. Discussion

This is the first study to accurately map prostate calcification in patients with prostate cancer using computational methods to analyze rich imaging data available from contemporaneous mpMRI and CT. Our study has shown a few important differences in the distribution of calcification compared to previous studies. Although calcification occurred more in the transition zone, there were a significant number in the peripheral zone (35%), a greater proportion than previously reported, for instance 17% [11] and 6.8% [12].

A higher incidence in the peripheral zone could be explained by differences in the patient cohort studied compared to other studies. This cohort had a high percentage of high-risk disease and history of previous treatment. As the majority of prostate cancers occur in the peripheral zone and calcification can be associated with cancer, this may explain the higher incidence in our cohort. The densities of the calcifications ranged from 133 to 1,966 HU, with a mean of 227 HU. This is comparable to the densities reported in previous studies conducted on smaller patient cohorts [3,17]. The volume of calcifications ranged from 4.8 to 1,263.6 mm^3. The larger foci were found more in the transition zone, consistent with previous studies.

An important finding of this study is that prostatic calcification can commonly occur within and in the locale of prostate cancer. In 12 patients, foci of calcification were within MRI-visible tumors. The presence of tumor calcification in this cohort is higher than previously observed [11]. This higher incidence may be explained again by many patients in this cohort having previous treatments and then having a local recurrence. We hypothesize that previous treatments such as radiotherapy or thermal ablation cause inflammation resulting in a healing response which leads to deposition of calcification. This process is seen in other organs such as the liver and kidneys [18,19] and has been reported after radiotherapy and thermal ablation in the prostate [20,21]. Furthermore, we found that in 24 patients, there were calcifications within 9 mm of the tumor, which is the ablation margin recommended for focal therapy [16].

The prostatic urethra is an important structure to protect in prostate therapies. Our analysis showed that in 13 patients calcification was in a periurethral distribution, and in 9 patients, calcifications were located between the urethra and tumor (see Fig. 1B). The presence of high-density material such as calcification in the prostate has been shown to cause aberration of ultrasound waves and photon attenuation in radiotherapy. These effects can cause significant differences in treatment dose for both ultrasound ablation and radiotherapy. For transurethral ultrasound ablation, for example, calcifications located around the urethra, between the urethra and tumor, or in the tumor itself, may lie in the path of the beam. If the presence of these calcifications is not accounted for in treatment planning, then there could be a risk of undertreatment and subsequent recurrence. Further studies are needed to model the effects of prostate calcification in treatment delivery in order to determine strategies and robust thresholds for treatment.

MRI has become a key imaging modality in the assessment of prostate cancer but calcifications are difficult to visualize in standard multiparametric protocols [22]. It is widely used to plan thermal ablation treatments such as HIFU, cryotherapy, and transurethral ultrasound ablation. However calcifications are often not visible on MRI and not routinely commented on in radiological reports. Therefore, the impact of calcification in these therapies is likely under-recognized and under-reported. In contrast, for patients undergoing radiotherapy, CT imaging is usually available and calcifications can be used as pseudofiducial markers to plan treatment [23]. However, most CT reports do not mention prostatic calcification, even though studies have shown an impact in dose delivery [3].

5. Conclusions

In this study, the location and density of prostatic calcifications were accurately mapped. The study has shown that prostatic calcifications are common in patients with prostate cancer. A large proportion of calcifications occur in and around tumors which could have an impact on their subsequent treatment.

DR.ENQI

Raw Herbal Compounds
PRODUCT GUIDE

Detox Kit:

Kemeluminescence -
NRF2, YEAST, FUNGUS, FAT SUPPORT;
Bladderwrack, Yarrow, Cascara Sagrada, Moss, Happy Tree, Madagascar, Periwinkle, Mayapple, Pacific Yew, Cloves, Amla, Coriander, Black Walnut, Kelp, White Pine Bark, Horny Goat Weed, Milk Thistle, Tribulus, Bitter Melon, Chaste Berry, African Pygeum, Cinnamon, Gynesylvestre, Hemp, Pau D Arco, African Bird Pepper, Cinchona Bark, Chinese Senega Root, Biden Pilosa, Houttuynia, Licorice, Skullcap, Scute Root, Ginseng, Rehmania, Er Bu Shir Tao, Bugleweed

Swadj Momatomix -
Marrow & Electromagnetism Support / Rich in Hydrogen, Phosphorus, Aromatic Amino Acid Phosphorus, Nettles, Wild Lettuce, Hydrogen, Plant Enzyme, &Alkaloid+ MATRIX

Antiviral Kit -

Antiviral
Antifungal
Antibacterial
mtDNA Protector
The most comprehensive organic antiviral kit ever assembled to fight viral infection and improve recovery

Antivirals -
Exogenous & Endogenous Pathogen Support
Cilantro, Celery, Chaparral, Olive Leaf, Oregano Leaf, Black Walnut, Lysine, Tyrosine, Thyme, Cleavers, Hyssop, Bladderwrack, Ginger

Antiviral Nutrient -
Pathogen Suppression Support
Manganese, Rosemary, Hydrangea, Bilberry, Rhizome Rei

Antiviral Oil -
Immunglobulin & Antibody Support
Oregano, Peppermint, Tea Tree, Cinnamon, Hyssop, Thyme, Clove, Ginger

Calcium -
Muscle & Bone Support
Blood Pressure, Insulin Control, Nerve Function, Muscle Contraction
Kelp, Calcium, Sesame, Cloves

Chromium & Vanadium -

Glucose Tolerance Factor & Eyesight Support
Fat Loss , Insulin Metabolism , Hydration , Muscle Integrity , Energy
Chromium, Fenugreek, Vanadium, Bitter Melon, Gymnema Sylvestre

Copper -
Pigment System Support
Cardiovascular Key, Heart Beat Nutrient, White Blood Cell Reg
Copper, Cilantro, Cloves, Milk Thistle

Iron -
Heme & Magnetism Support
Electron Circulation, Digestive System, Thermogenesis, Brain Power
Iron, Yellow Dock, Stinging Nettles, Chaparral

Magnesium -
Energy & Light Metabolism Support
Muscle Function, Energy, Builds ; Proteins/ Enzymes/ Hormones , DNA Repair
Blue Vervain, Burdock, Parsley, Magnesium

Muscle Drip -
Children/Adults Multivitamin & Bone Tendon Compound
Blood Oxygen, Breakdown Lactic Acid, Builds Blood Cells Faster, Cleans Lymphatic System
Elderberries, Cherries, Sea Moss, Stinging Nettles, Horsetail, Lily of the Valley, Bladderwrack, Bromide,

Melatonin, Phosphorus, Boron, Calcium, Strontium

Muscle Plants -
Children + Adults Multivitamin & Muscle/Joint Compound
Gout, Autography, Enhanced Healing, Arthritis, Remove Stones
Elderberries, Cherries, Bugleweed, Hombre Grande, Blue Vervain, Chaparral, Ginseng, Rhodiola, Boswellia, Eluethero, Melatonin, Phosphorus, Magnesium

Selenium -
Immune Plasma Support
Thyroid Health, Cancer Suppression, Mental Health, Tumor Suppression
Selenium, Burdock, Bladderwrack, Sarsaparilla

Swadj Momatomix -
Marrow & Electromagnetism Support / Rich in Hydrogen, Phosphorus, Aromatic Amino Acid
Phosphorus, Nettles, Wild Lettuce, Hydrogen, Plant Enzyme, &Alkaloid+ MATRIX

Zinc -
Skin & Enzyme Support
Anabolic Boost, Immune System Nutrient, Stem Cell Health, Gene Support
Rosemary, Chlorella, Sage, Zinc

Watermelanin -
Nootropic, Dopamine, Muscle Recovery, Nourish

Your Pineal Gland, DMT Support
Raw Organic Non-GMO Black Watermelon Seeds
Lupulin

Anabolic Hormone Help -
Anabolic Hormones, AMPK & Circadian Support
Jiaogulan, Wild Lettuce, Tribulus, Longjack, Maca &
Pollen Blend

Histonic -
Histone Sirtuin Support
Grape Skin, Resveratrol, Tyrosine Analogue, Japanese
Knotweed

Ocean Steak -
Vegan B12, Carbon, Nucleoside, Protein, Nucleotide,
Omega 3 & Eye Support
Phytoplankton, Duckweed, Chlorella, Purple Laver,
Chondrus Crispus & C60 Lutein, Zeaxanthin, Ocean
Pigment Matrix

Chrondris Crispus -
Structured Water Mucus Membrane Support
Copper, Cilantro, Cloves, Milk Thistle

NON GMO Moringa -
Whole Body Nutrition Support
Raw Organic Non-GMO Moringa

Purple Phaze -
Anti-Aging Longevity Support
FoTi, Pumpkin Seed, NMN, Bhringaraj, Biotin, Silica,
Tyrosine, Yucca, White Willow Bark, French Lilac,

NAD

Every item on this list, every compound is not only from God but works on the skin from the inside out, what we need now is topical.

Topical = Tropical

Batana is Great but it's expensive and incomplete.

Researchers identify 135 new melanin genes responsible for pigmentation

Date: August 11, 2023

Source: University of Oklahoma

Summary: The skin, hair and eye color of more than eight billion humans is determined by the light-absorbing pigment known as melanin. New research has identified 135 new genes associated with pigmentation. Vitamin D and Vitamin A... I told you nature doesn't wait to be discovered before getting to work! Melanin vs Diabetes as a Ministry & Movement isn't waiting around to save lives... We have saving lives and creating thought leaders for 20 years!!! The thing is science just discovered 135 genes for pigment and melanin, how the F@3$ have the been acting as if.... This is why we rely on Nature, God & our Ancestors.

We are teaching the world, showing the world...

#HealingLooksLikeThis

Most people don't know what the process of Healing actually Looks Like!!!

People judge health by how your skin looks, literally your complexion. Your Complex of Ions!

Complexion - the general aspect or character of something; the natural color, texture, and appearance of a person's skin, especially of the face.

complexion (n.)
mid-14c., complexioun, "temperament, natural disposition of body or mind," from Old French complexion, complession "**combination of humors**," hence "temperament, character, make-up," from Latin complexionem (nominative complexio) "combination" (in Late Latin, "physical constitution"), from complexus "surrounding, encompassing," past participle of complecti "to encircle, embrace," in transferred use, "to hold fast, master, comprehend," from com "with, together" (see com-) + plectere "to weave, braid, twine, entwine," from PIE *plek-to-, suffixed form of root *plek- "to plait."
The Middle English sense is from the old medicine notion of bodily constitution or general nature resulting from blending of the four primary qualities (hot, cold, dry, moist) or humors (blood, phlegm, choler, black choler). The specific meaning

"**<u>color or hue of the skin of the face</u>**" developed by mid-15c. In medieval physiology, the color of the face was believed to be caused by the balance of humors in the body and indicate temperament or health. The word rarely is used in the sense of "state of being complex."
also from mid-14c.

Humor - the quality of being amusing or comic, especially as expressed in literature or speech; a mood or state of mind. **Each of the four chief fluids of the body (blood, phlegm, yellow bile (choler), and black bile (melancholy)) that were thought to determine a person's physical and mental qualities** by the relative proportions in which they were present.

humor (n.)
mid-14c., "**fluid or juice of an animal or plant**," from Old North French humour "liquid, dampness; (medical) humor" (Old French humor, umor; Modern French humeur), from Latin umor "body fluid" (also humor, by false association with **humus "earth"**); related to umere "**be wet**, moist," and to uvescere "become wet" (see humid).
In old medicine, "any of the four body fluids" (blood, phlegm, choler, and melancholy or black bile).

*The human body had four humors—blood, phlegm, yellow bile, and black bile—which, in turn, were associated with particular organs. Blood came from the heart, phlegm from the brain, yellow bile from the liver, and black bile from the spleen. Galen and Avicenna attributed certain elemental qualities to each humor. Blood was hot and moist, like air; phlegm was cold and moist, like water; yellow bile was hot and dry, like fire; and black bile was cold and dry, like earth. In effect, the human body was a microcosm of the larger world. [Robert S. Gottfried, "The Black Death," 1983]

Their relative proportions were thought to determine physical condition and state of mind. This gave humor an extended sense of "mood, temporary state of mind" (recorded from 1520s); the sense of "amusing quality, funniness, jocular turn of mind" is first recorded 1680s, probably via sense of "whim, caprice" as determined by state of mind (1560s), which also produced the verb sense of "indulge (someone's) fancy or disposition." Modern French has them as doublets: humeur "disposition, mood, whim;" humour "humor." "The pronunciation of the initial h is only of recent date, and is sometimes omitted ..." [OED].

For aid in distinguishing the various devices that tend to be grouped under "humor," this guide, from Henry W. Fowler ["Modern English Usage," 1926] may be of use:

HUMOR: motive/aim: discovery; province: human nature; method/means: observation; audience: the sympathetic

WIT: motive/aim: throwing light; province: words & ideas; method/means: surprise; audience: the intelligent

SATIRE: motive/aim: amendment; province: morals & manners; method/means: accentuation; audience: the self-satisfied

SARCASM: motive/aim: inflicting pain; province: faults & foibles; method/means: inversion; audience: victim & bystander

INVECTIVE: motive/aim: discredit; province: misconduct; method/means: direct statement; audience: the public

IRONY: motive/aim: exclusiveness; province: statement of facts; method/means: mystification; audience: an inner circle

CYNICISM: motive/aim: self-justification; province: morals; method/means: exposure of nakedness; audience: the respectable

SARDONIC: motive/aim: self-relief; province: adversity; method/means: pessimism; audience: the self

also from mid-14c.

We alway have to remember the Greeks were educated by the Egyptians, ie…

Eu - Good, Perfect, Complete

Melanin (Melanos) - Black

EuMelanin is the new way to reference Osiris.

The new usage of humor came from state of mind, which came from your health, based in the balance of fluids.

#StayWet

The herbs and bitters are to condition the internal fluids, the BleuMagick conditions the body's waters, we are now going to top it off with #SkinFood, to make sure you can #StayWet.

Please read &/or reread Lymphatic Immunity, Mitochondria Water, HydroChemistry...

You've got to learn everything you can from these books about Water. Then you will be ready to apply these principles and practices, Kitchen Chemistry, Orthorexia & this book espouse! Truth be told, these 3 books are plug and play immediately... but the further study is what refines you. You have to disappear sometime and come back stronger. You don't that by consuming new information in your absence.

The biggest difference between those in the Rat Race, and those who aren't, is Priority of Consuming New Information. Reading.

What does it mean to you that, the other pigments in the skin control Melanin production?

What does it mean to you that, they just discovered 3000 new types of Neurons?

Neurons are either specialized Melanocytes or Melanocytes are specialized Neurons, they have discovered 3,000 new types Naga.... Wake Up!!! Either your whole body is a Brain or a Heart! The Heart has all of these cells, Neurons, Nerves, Melanocytes etc...

What does it mean to you that, they just discovered 135 genes that are associated with Pigment? Is that 135 genes for the Skin? Brain? Heart???

My goal is to make #SkinFood inexpensive enough for you and your family to use twice a day, that way we can #StayWet.

In L'Goat we explain in detail how water builds what it needs, with the right conditions. First thing is well, Water. Second thing obviously is Retinoids, to fertilize the soil. Then of course Sunlight...

You are the Dust of the Ground, Divine Soil, remember that the ground exerts pressure on seeds. You need the proper exercise, to create that mechanical pressure to stimulate growth and regeneration. Mechanical Pressure helps to circulate Magnetism, this is the #BleuMagick of #ElectroMagneticTissue.

If this is your first book of ours that you have read... God Bless Eu, or maybe this isn't your first book but you haven't read PiezoElectroChemistry, please do that...

You are the Fruit of Melanin, your S.elf O.rganizing U.niversal L.ight.

Soul is the Fruit of PhotoVoltaic Pigment.

The Bible has many allusions to the **Sun** and its 12 houses, but they replace the Sun with the Son. The Bible is full of Truth, full of Science, you just have to know what your looking at. Kemetic Science is a mixture of Photochemistry, Photobiology & Acoustics. The key is remembering that Light and Sound only exist in your mind. The electromagnetic spectrum you are used to seeing is deceptive, so I have taken the liberty to provide you with a more straight forward version in this book.

ElectronVolts - an electronvolt (symbol eV, also written electron-volt and electron volt) is the measure of an amount of_**kinetic energy** gained by a single electron accelerating from rest through an electric potential difference of one volt in vacuum, 1 eV equal to the exact value 1.602176634×10−19 J, a unit of energy or work, **the work** **required to move an electron** through a potential difference of one volt. 1 eV would correspond to an infrared photon of wavelength 1240 nm or frequency 241.8 THz.

4-12 ELECTRON VOLTS = UVC 100-320 NM DEATH WM

3.9 ELECTRON VOLTS = UVB SKIN 290-320 NM

DISEASE JW

3.4 ELECTRON VOLTS = UVA 320-400 NM EYE DISEASE SW

.001 ELECTRON VOLTS = FAR INFRARED 1000000 NM BEYOND THIS POINT IS RADIO WAVES

.4 ELECTRON VOLTS = NEAR FAR INFRARED 3000 NM

.8 ELECTRON VOLTS = MEDIUM INFRARED 1500 NM

1.5 ELECTRON VOLTS = NEAR INFRARED 780 NM

1.7 ELECTRON VOLTS = VISIBLE RED 620-780 NM

2 ELECTRON VOLTS = VISIBLE ORANGE 585-620 NM

2.1 ELECTRON VOLTS = VISIBLE YELLOW 570-585 NM

2.3 ELECTRON VOLTS = VISIBLE GREEN 490-570 NM

2.6 ELECTRON VOLTS = VISIBLE BLUE 440-490 NM

2.9 ELECTRON VOLTS = VISIBLE INDIGO 420-440 NM

3 ELECTRON VOLTS = VISIBLE VIOLET 400-420 NM

We will look at the E.M. Spectrum in terms of Electron Volts, this makes more sense because all of chemistry is based on the movement of electrons. The Sun is the great visible agent of the first cause. This of course means you have to rethink the whole entire ElectroChemistry aka Dr. Sebi vs Dr. EnQi book…

Sound Range: 20 to 20,000 Hz

Voice Range 90 to 255 Hz

Radio Range: 1 hertz up to 3,000 billion hertz. Below Radio is Cellular, Extremely low frequency (ELF) electric and magnetic fields (EMF) occupy the lower part of the electromagnetic spectrum in the frequency range 0-100 kHz. ELF EMF result from electrically charged particles.

Infrared Range 1 Trillion Hertz to … this is where our body heat is…

TECHNOLOGY EQUIPMENT RECAP

<u>HydroGenes</u> - 1! Proton and 1! Electron.

<u>Melanocytes</u> - Photovoltaic Cells

<u>Neurons/Nerves</u> - Electromagnetic Cells

<u>Fascia</u> - Plasma Medium (misonomered Ether)

<u>Brain</u> - CPU, Inductor

<u>Brainstem</u> - Two-way Adapter for CPU into the Motherboard

<u>Pineal Gland</u> - Receiver, Crystal Tuner & Actuator Arm/Head responsible for Phosphorescence, Thermoluminescence, Piezoelectricity, Birefringence & Harmonic Generation (very much like the otoconia in the ears)

<u>Operating System</u> - Deductive Logic or PQ

<u>Heart</u> - Hydraulic Ram, Turbine (from the Greek τύρβη, tyrbē, or Latin turbo, meaning vortex) and Hard Drive.

<u>Melanosomes</u> - Alternators

<u>Mitochondria</u> - Motors

<u>Myelin Sheath</u> - Insulation

<u>Cytoskeleton</u> - Filaments

<u>Phospholipids</u> - Capacitors, Dielectric Material (lipids in general)

<u>Spine</u> - Piezoelectric, Motherboard, Radio Wave Antenna

<u>RBC</u> - Floppy Discs

<u>Lymph Nodes</u> - Filters, Nodes

<u>Tastebuds</u> - Electronic Scanners

<u>Protein</u> - Transformer

<u>Transformers 'Roll Out'</u> - Conformational Change (Macromolecule Shape Shifting)

<u>Antioxidants</u> - Semi-conductors (especially the selenium based...)

<u>Body Cells</u> - Plasma based Crystal disc, fitted with integrated circuits as well as gates and channels (see Human Cell Membrane and/or Computer Chip)

<u>Nerves & Vessels</u> - 'Copper' wires (CoAxial Cables) and Fiber Optics

<u>Pigment, Nerve & Blood Clusters</u> - Input Devices like a Mouse, Keyboard, etc...

<u>DNA</u> - Piezoelectric, Antenna, Data Storing Inductors.

DNA sub entry **<u>Tissues</u>** - Short Living Stories.

DNA sub entry **<u>Genome</u>** - Substrate & Product, a digital Library (HardDrive) of all your Ancestors have ever seen, said, touched, tasted or heard.

DNA sub entry **<u>Chromosome</u>** - Rewritable Unlimited Storage Books (Folders) of the Library, DNA.

DNA sub entry **<u>Histone</u>** - Writing instrument, encoders and **book spines**.

DNA sub entry **<u>non-coding RNA</u>** - Self Organizing Books Shelves

DNA sub entry **<u>Gene</u>** - Chapters (Files) in the Books, source codes.

DNA sub entry **<u>Messenger RNA</u>** - Protein Information, a Sentence.

DNA sub entry **<u>Codon</u>** - Word (Binary Code there are 2 bonds between each 3 nucleotides representing their arrangement), Amino Acid.

DNA sub entry **Nucleotide** - Letter

DNA sub entry **Nucleoside** - Bits of Information

Collagen Based Tissue - Piezoelectric Inductors

Stomach - Chemical Mixer

Lumen - the SI unit of luminous flux = to the amount of light emitted per second..... or hollow structures in vessels and cells... hmmm????

Eyes - Camera Lens/Charge Coupled Device (CCD), Digital to Analogue Converter, Complex Photovoltaic Cells/Photodetector...

Amino Acids - Fuses that can be almost anything!

Nucleic Acid - Actual Intelligence (self powering too).

N-Type Semiconductors - Selenium or Silica doped with Phosphorus (Alkaline-ish)

P-Type Semiconductors - Selenium or Silica doped with Boron (Acid-ish)

PN Junction - <u>Crystal Lattice Structure</u> Material allowing the flowing of electrons in one direction.

Bone and Fascia seem to be a massive N-Type, P-Type, PN Junction Super computer on it's own... especially if we add in the Piezoelectricity & Vitamin D!

<u>Rectifier</u> - N-Type + P-Type + PN Junction in Bone

<u>Melanin</u> - CPU Core, Solar Repeater

<u>Human Cell Membrane and/or Computer Chip</u> - A flat semiconducting (crystal) disc or wafer, with integrated circuits (resistors/conductors) and/or gates & channels. We now have to add the filaments into this Crystal Disc we call a Body Cell or Somatic Cell.

<u>Transistors</u> - a semiconductor device with three connections, capable of amplification in addition to rectification.

The location that a virus goes viral in, is called a **<u>Hotspot</u>**? WTH!

<u>Virus</u> - an infective agent that typically consists of a nucleic acid molecule in a protein coat, is too small to be seen by light microscopy, and is able to multiply only within the living cells of a host.

Wait you see that, it is happening again! Host...

See look there is another definition of **<u>Virus</u>** - a piece of code that is capable of copying itself and typically has a detrimental effect, such as corrupting the system or destroying data.

Wait a damn minute! DNA is a piece of **<u>code</u>**... A viral strand of DNA or RNA that can jump host is fully capable in that context of copying itself, one would even argue, that is it's only 'motion'. The detrimental effects of corrupting the system (physical illness) or destroying data (mental illness), can clearly be seen anthropomorphically.

Alien - Virus

Culture - the arts and other manifestations of human intellectual achievement regarded collectively, the customs, arts, social institutions, and achievements of a particular nation, people, or other social group. The cultivation of bacteria, tissue cells, etc. in an artificial medium containing nutrients, a preparation of cells obtained from a culture. The cultivation of **plants**.

Going Live - become operational.

Live Stream - a live transmission of an event over the internet, transmit or receive live video and audio coverage of (an event) over the internet.

The Web - Arachnoid Mater

Download - copy (data) from one computer system to another, typically over the internet, an act or process of downloading data.

Upload - transfer (data) from one computer to another, typically to one that is larger or remote from the user or functioning as a server, an act or process of downloading data.

<u>Data</u> - facts and statistics collected together for reference or analysis; the quantities, characters, or symbols on which operations are performed by a computer, being stored and transmitted in the form of electrical signals and recorded on magnetic, optical, or mechanical recording media.

<u>Host</u> - an animal or plant on or in which a parasite or commensal organism lives. VS

<u>Host</u> - store (a website or other data) on a server or other computer so that it can be accessed over the internet.

<u>Transmission</u> is the act of transferring something from one spot to another, like a radio or TV broadcast, or a disease going from one person to another.

I am highlighting the unknown and proposing we may have some answers! <u>Infection - an infectious disease.</u>

plural noun: infections "a chest infection"

Vs

<u>Infection</u> - the presence of a virus in, or its introduction into, a computer system. What is a computer system?

<u>Computer System</u> - a computer system is a programmable electronic device that can accept input; store data; and retrieve, process and output information.

<u>Pandemic language = Virology/Biology language.</u> The question is, why? The next question is what does that have to do with Dr. Sebi or Robert Becker? The obvious....

<u>Computer System</u> - a computer system is a programmable electronic device that can accept input; store data; and retrieve, process and output information.

<u>Computer System</u> - a single information processor but usually a group of processors that have specified and general computations; grouped by hardware ie... liver cells, lung cells, brain cells etc.. What you think?

<u>Exercise</u> - activity requiring physical effort, carried out to sustain or improve health and fitness. "exercise improves your heart and lung power"

<u>Exercise</u> - computer training or computer based training.

<u>Exigenetics</u> - Term created by Dr. EnQi for Melanin vs Diabetes research, denoting the control that exercise has over gene expression.

<u>Hydration</u> - the process of inducing gelling, ionizing, dissolution & turbulent flow with activation of cytochrome c (via infrared light).

<u>Resonance</u> - the quality in a sound of being deep, full, and reverberating. "the resonance of his voice"

- The ability to evoke or suggest images, memories, and emotions."the concepts lose their emotional resonance"

- The reinforcement or prolongation of sound by reflection from a surface or by the synchronous vibration of a neighboring object.

- The condition in which an electric circuit or device produces the largest possible response to an applied oscillating signal, especially when its inductive and its capacitative reactances are balanced.

- The condition in which an object or system is subjected to an oscillating force having a frequency close to its own natural frequency.

- The occurrence of a simple ratio between the periods of revolution of two bodies about a single primary.

- The state attributed to certain molecules of having a structure that cannot adequately be represented by a single structural formula but is a composite of two or more structures of higher energy.

- • A short-lived subatomic particle that is an excited state of a more stable particle.

Induction - the action or process of inducting someone to a position or organization."the league's induction into the Baseball Hall of Fame"

Induction - a formal introduction to a new job or position.plural noun: inductions
"an induction course"
enlistment into military service.

Induction - The process or action of bringing about or giving rise to something."isolation, starvation, and other forms of stress induction" the process of bringing on childbirth or abortion by artificial means, typically by the use of drugs.

Induction - The inference of a general law from particular instances.

Induction -"the admission that laws of nature cannot be established by induction" the production of facts to prove a general statement.

Induction - a means of proving a theorem by showing that if it is true of any particular case it is true of the next case in a series, and then showing that it is indeed true in one particular case.

Induction - noun: mathematical induction; plural noun: mathematicals inductionthe production of an electric or magnetic state by the proximity (without contact) of an electrified or magnetized body.

Induction - The production of an electric current in a conductor by varying the magnetic field applied to the conductor.

Induction - The stage of the working cycle of an internal combustion engine in which the fuel mixture is drawn into the cylinders.

Is there anyone reading this that would disagree with our body fitting these definitions, the definitions of a computer?

Man this thought experiment just got a lot more interesting didn't it? MIT and the US Military are different types of receipts huh? Is it possible frequency resonance, spreads disease? Human modems? Can Shedding be a broadcast signal?

Wi-Fi is a wireless networking technology that uses radio waves to provide wireless high-speed Internet access. A common misconception is that the term **Wi-Fi** is short for "wireless fidelity," however Wi-Fi is a trademarked phrase that refers to IEEE 802.11x standards.

<u>Viral shedding</u> is a term for when viruses are replicating or reproducing, the virus is being led out of the host cell where it's replicating or

reproducing ... Viral shedding is the expulsion and release of virus progeny following successful reproduction during a host cell infection. Once replication has been completed and the host cell is exhausted of all resources in making viral progeny, the viruses may begin to leave the cell by several methods.

<u>Vaccine</u> - a substance used to stimulate immunity to a particular infectious disease or pathogen, typically prepared from

an inactivated or weakened form of the causative agent or from

its constituents or products.

<u>Vaccine</u> - a program designed to detect computer viruses and inactivate them.

"the rate of use of vaccines for computer viruses is not as high as in the US, Japan, and other countries"

<u>Application</u> - a medicinal substance put on the skin.

<u>Application</u> - a program or piece of software designed and written to fulfill a particular purpose of the user.

In our thought experiment, if a virus is simply the

media for harmful information...

<u>Media</u> - an intermediate layer in the wall of a blood vessel or lymphatic vessel.

<u>Media</u> - the main means of mass communication (broadcasting, publishing, and the internet) regarded collectively.

<u>DOPE</u> - an illicit drug (such as heroin or cocaine) used for its intoxicating or euphoric effects especially : MARIJUANA (dopamine altering)

<u>Dope</u> - a preparation (such as an anabolic steroid, diuretic, or tranquilizer) given to a racehorse to help or hinder its performance

<u>To Dope</u> - In semiconductor production, to dope is the intentional introduction of impurities into an intrinsic semiconductor for the purpose of modulating its electrical, optical and structural properties. The doped material is referred to as an extrinsic semiconductor.

<u>Short Circuit</u> - Cardiac Arrest?

<u>Short Circuit</u> - Multiple Sclerosis (due to loss of insulation)

<u>Overheating</u> - Fever?

<u>Overcurrent</u> - Inflammation

With Infection and Virus included we are onto

something.

Current - belonging to the present time; happening or being used or done now.

Current - a body of water or air moving in a *definite* direction, especially through a surrounding body of water or air in which there is less movement.

Current - a flow of electricity that results from the ordered directional movement of electrically charged particles.

Current - a quantity representing the rate of flow of electric charge, usually measured in amperes.

Current - the general tendency or course of events or opinion.

Leakage Current - the unintended loss of energy, gain of resistance or results of faulty/worn out insulation.

Plasma - Electric Currents or Electric Current Carrier

Electric Current - Magnetic Field (AtomSphere) Carrier

Alternating Magnetic & Electric Waves - Light

NeuroTransmitters - Record of ElectroMagnetic Waves produced by Neurons (ElectroChemical Message)

Hormones - Large simple versions of NeuroTransmitters (ElectroChemical Message)

Malware - External Negative Mental Programming

Food - Informative Electronic Batteries

0) Movement and sound create energy from water for basic cellular function, via the EnQi Cycle which includes Mitochondria Water. This system slowly increases as all other energy systems fail.

1) Phosphocreatine - anaerobic (no respiration required), phosphocreatine donates it "phospho" to ADP to recycle ATP. This makes 10 ATP per second, its a 1 to 1 ratio (1 phosphocreatine creates 1 ATP) and this is the jump start energy.

2) Anaerobic Glycolysis - anaerobic (no respiration required), Glycogen &/or Glucose to Lactate, 5 ATP per second, 1 to 3 ratio (1 Glycogen creates 3 ATP while 1 Glucose creates 2 ATP) and this is bulk of the energy we focus on, 9 - 120 seconds.

3) NAD/Cytochrome 1 - aerobic (requires oxygen), Glycogen &/or Glucose to CO_2/H_2O, 2.5 ATP per second, 1 to 38 ratio (1 Glycogen &/or Glucose creates 38 ATP), 2 minutes up to 2 hours.

4) FAD/Cytochrome 2 - aerobic (requires oxygen), FFA &/or Triglycerides to CO_2/H_2O, 1.5 ATP per second, 1 to 360 ratio (1 Glycogen &/or Glucose creates 360 ATP), 2 minutes up to 2 days.

Food rule of thumb - Resynthesis of ATP of Inverse to Yield, the closer the ratio is to 1:1 the fast it can be recycled.

Muscle rule of thumb - Frequently used muscle is slow twitch, Fast twitch is slowly used (at that's the blueprint).

Electric Power - the **rate** at which work is done or energy is transformed into an electrical circuit. Simply put, it is a measure of how much energy is used in a span of time.

Conductor - a person who directs the performance of an orchestra or choir.

Conductor - a material or device that conducts or transmits heat, electricity, or sound, especially when regarded in terms of its capacity to do this.

Lymphatic System - Watermill

Circulatory System - Generator

Integumentary System - Photovoltaic Diaphragm

Immune System - Antivirus, Malware Scanner, Frequency Filter & Rectifier

Nervous System - Power Transmission and Cellular Communications Lines

<u>Fascia System</u> - HydroElectric Grid, Scaffolding

<u>Respiratory System</u> - Windmill

<u>Windmill</u> - a structure that converts wind power or "air" power into rotational energy or vortex energy, to mill grain. In our case grain is Magnetism!

MAGNETS ARE DEFINED BY GRAINS
MAGNETIC GRAINS ARE DEFINED BY APPLIED
STRESS AND CRYSTAL GEOMETRY
SPM SUPERMAGNETIC
SD SINGLE DOMAIN
PSD PSEUDO DOMAIN
MD MULTIDOMAIN

<u>Reproductive System</u> - Quine (self-replicating programs)

<u>Skeletal System</u> - Piezoelectric Crystal Shaped to produced highly specific frequency under stress, Dynamic Oscillators.

<u>Urinary System</u> - Industrial Wastewater, Return Flow, Surface Runoff, Urban Runoff Agricultural & Animal Husbandry Wastewater

<u>Digestive System</u> - Massive Inductor

<u>Mouth</u> - Industrial Grinder

<u>Endocrine System</u> - Programmer for Human Cell Membrane and/or Crystal Gel Computer Chips

<u>Human Being</u> - Resonator

<u>Vessels</u> - Pipes

<u>Aromatic Ring</u> - Cyclotron (Particle Accelerator)

<u>Glycation</u> - Corrosion

<u>Exegenetics</u> - Holistic Biomechanics; the purposeful science of combining light, water, diet & exercise to effect DNA.

<u>EnQi's 1st Law of Metabolism</u> - The conversion rate of cholesterol should match the activity of Melanin in the skin. These two systems are designed to be and stay coupled. A dark skin person with low sunlight intake and low exercise is going to die from a Metabolic Complication. The only time Animal Flesh is safe to be consumed by a Eumelanin Dominant person is in times of starvation or extremely high activity.

This Law is a Constant and when broken results in disease every time.

<u>EnQi's 2nD Law of Metabolism</u> - The average rate of applied mechanical stress on the bone electrically stimulating bone marrow, determines the rate of bone deterioration and Red Blood Cell production.

<u>EnQi's 3rd Law of Metabolism</u> - The human body metabolizes Transverse Waves and Mechanical Waves into Electricity. Electricity is the main driver of Biochemistry. Exercise is just as potent a driver of Biochemistry as the Sun.

EnQi's 4th Law of Metabolism - Electron movement and bonding is the Nature of Chemistry. PhotoChemistry and PiezoElectroChemistry are the Primary drivers of Biochemistry.

The Ancients discovered this and created Martial Artforms as a way to clean the Bone, Bone Marrow & Brain. Plaque & Sugar are the top drivers of Brain Disease. The things destroying the Heart are secondarily destroying the brain, and they are the breaking of these Universal Laws.

EnQi's 5th Law of Metabolism - Nutrients are actually substrates that must be transformed via biochemistry to be meaningful. This means that providing your body with lots of nutrition without the Water, Light & Exercise don't work alone.

EnQi's 6th Law of Metabolism - The Body maintains the least amount of bone marrow required to handle blood demand. The marrow is very energy demanding, thus attracting and storing fat for energy, eventually becoming fat itself. Fatty bone marrow is called yellow bone marrow. Yellow Bone Marrow can be reconverted to Red Bone Marrow should the body's demands require it, and the body's resources facilitate it. The primary driver is pressure, hormesis training on the Bones. BMR is heavily driven by Bone Marrow, this means Bone Marrow is a driver if insulin and insulin resistance.

<u>EnQi's 7th Law of Metabolism</u> - The system of pigments throughout the body are for metabolism of Light, actual Soulfood. The Adsorption & Absorption of Photons by Water.

Adsorption - increase in the concentration of a dissolved substance at the interface of a condensed and a liquid phase due to the operation of surface forces.

Absorption - a physical or chemical phenomenon or a process in which atoms, molecules or ions enter some bulk phase – liquid or solid material. This is a different process from adsorption, since molecules undergoing absorption are taken up by the volume, not by the surface.

<u>EnQi's 8th Law of Metabolism</u> - in a diabetic state, sugar is simply invisible to the body. Sugar is not being "sensed" because it's not being converted to energy. In this state of starvation the body turns on every pathway it has to produce sugar from everything you have in your body, fats and proteins included.

This is the reason that it seems like no matter what you eat or 'don't eat', your blood sugar goes up. It's very frustrating. The only way to make it stop is converting that substrate (glucose) into it's final product (energy). The reception of the actual energy, tells the body to stop producing substrate, we good. This must start in the legs and back, the largest muscles but most overlooked. The legs are particularly punished by sitting for extended periods of time, 3-6 hours straight, for a total over 3/4 the time your awake! The leg circulation atrophies and destroys the nerves, nerves are neurons that need a lot of nutrients!

*You must cross reference any and all protocols; food, exercise, medication etc... with the Constitution book & Declaration of Independence!

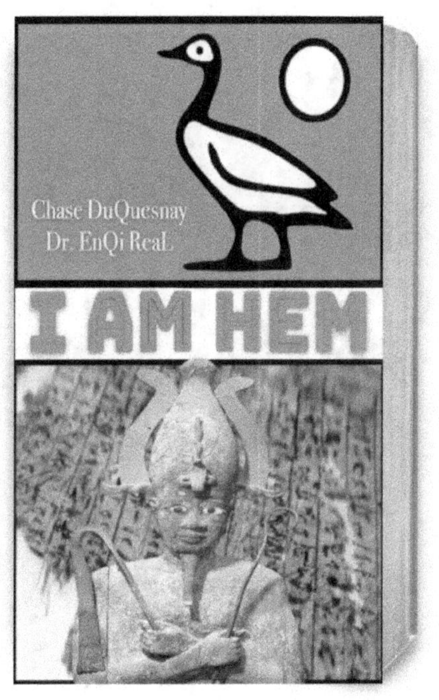

Chase DuQuesnay
Dr. EnQi ReaL
I AM HEM

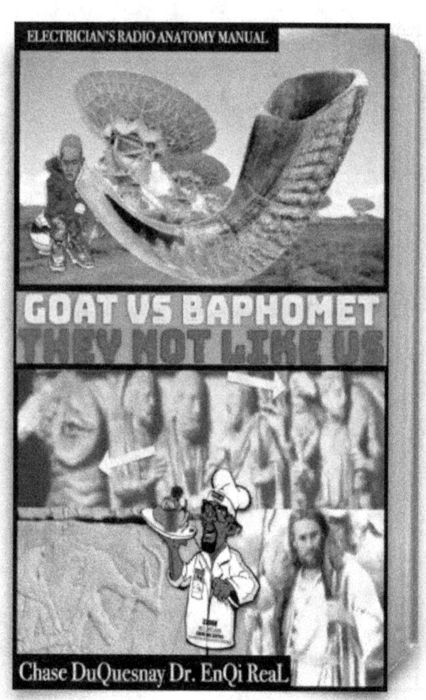

ELECTRICIAN'S RADIO ANATOMY MANUAL
GOAT VS BAPHOMET
THEY NOT LIKE US
Chase DuQuesnay Dr. EnQi ReaL

www.ingramcontent.com/pod-product-compliance
Lightning Source LLC
Chambersburg PA
CBHW071027250726
48653CB00005B/1753